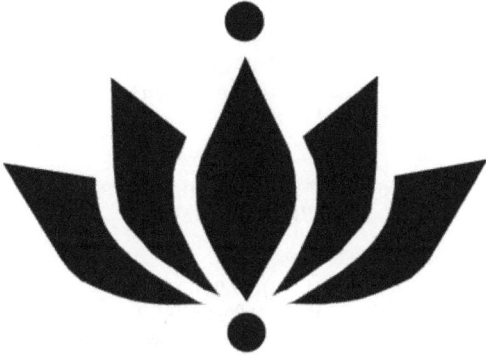

"Without love,
without humor,
Yoga is just
a lot of hard work."
                    - <u>Steve Ross</u>

This is a work of comedy. All quotes, statements, and jokes in this book are based on humor and parody, and any resemblance to real people or incidents is purely coincidental.

YOGA LAFFS
Compiled & Edited by Mike Callie & Laurence Berkley

Published by
HILARIOUS Press
5470 Birchbrook Court
Las Vegas, Nevada
89120

ISBN 13: 978-0-9646820-5-4
ISBN 10: 0-9646820-5-2
Library of Congress Control Number: 2013905082

Text set in Algerian
Book cover design and interior layout by
Crescent Moon Design Studio
www.cmds.co

Printed in the USA
First printing – HILARIOUS Press edition – March 2013

10 9 8 7 6 5 4 3 2 1

Visit our web site at
www.yogalaffs.com

SPECIAL FIRST EDITION PRINTING

YOGA LAFFS

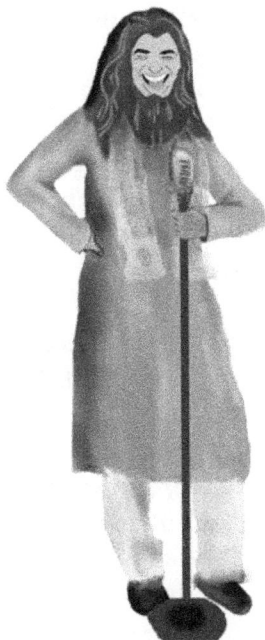

THE LAUGHTER OF YOGA

Edited & Compiled By:
Mike Callie & Laurence Berkley
Published By:

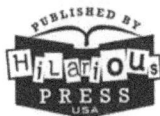

PUBLISHED BY
Hilarious
PRESS
USA

yogalaffs.com

MEET THE AUTHORS

MIKE CALLIE, a television and motion picture comedy writer, has been making America laugh for over 40 years. He has written several joke books and has provided special comedy material for top comedians and TV comedy shows and specials as well as being the creator, writer and producer of two of the funniest "Joke Movies" in history: *If You Don't Stop It...You'll Go Blind!!!* and its sequel, *Can I Do It 'Til I need Glasses?* which collectively grossed over $50 million in the 1970s and 1980s in box office and video sales/rentals.

Callie, one of the movers and shakers of the Comedy Club Boom of the 1980s (his 'Laff Stop' Comedy Clubs had over 10 locations throughout the U.S.), is a world renowned joke authority and joke book collector, along with being a recognized aficionado of all things comedy. He has over 5,400 joke books (and counting) in his personal collection; only the Library of Congress has more.

Callie currently resides in his underpriced Paradise Springs home in Las Vegas where he can personally guide the physical fitness and behavioral training of his loving and contrary son, Jack.

MEET THE AUTHORS

LAURENCE BERKLEY has been a student and teacher of Hatha Yoga for over 45 years and still going strong.

He began his studies and training in Southern California and has taught the Yoga arts in Europe, Asia, and throughout the United States.

In addition, Laurence also taught and trained in all aspects of the Martial Arts, and has attained the ranking of 5th degree Black Belt status while integrating the principles and disciplines of the Martial Arts into his personalized style of Yoga training.

The ancient studies have been an important part of his Yoga as well as today's Yoga disciplines, where Mr. Berkley combines music, humor, and the performing arts dance into his Yoga classes, which he conducts in Nevada and California with his associate, Ms. Jean Nix.

Mr. Berkley has 5 children and 11 grandchildren. His passion for Martial Arts, dance and laughter are the inspirations for his Yoga.

This book is a testament to that.[1]

---

[1] *It should be noted that Callie & Berkley are not only close personal friends and literary collaborators, but, according to recent police and Red Cross DNA tests, they are also blood cousins.*

A SPECIAL THANK YOU....

The Authors would like to thank all the many current and former Yoga Students, Teachers and Fans for their invaluable contributions and wonderful sense of humor in the publication of YOGA LAFFS.

We would also like to thank: Biff Manard; Richard Mc Swain, Hometown Digitals; Charity Luthy, Crescent Moon Design Studio; Dr. Thomas Parisi; Dr. Dan Walsh; Jack Callie; Miriam Field; Jorn Rossi; and Paul Krause for their encouragement and professional assistance to make "The World's First Yoga Humor Book" possible.

Thank You,
Mike Callie & Laurence Berkley

PREFACE

"Life would be tragic, but for our capacity to laugh at ourselves."

Maharishi Mahesh Yogi in a conversation with the Beatles as recalled by John Lennon – Rishikesh, India, 1968

For many hundreds of years In India and Tibet, Yoga humor was a special tradition and a unique way of expressing the study of Yoga.

The ancient Yoga teachers Milarepa (1040-1123 C.E.) and Drukpa (1455-1570 C.E) were prominent Yoga Masters who taught Yoga through humor, poems, songs and dance. One in particular, Swami Akkulkot, was a serious Yogi and an enlightened teacher who liked to laugh and used the humorous and "crazy wisdom" of that tradition in his teachings. He was considered like "the swan who flies freely from pond to pond enjoying himself as he laughed and sang" while teaching the joys and wisdom of Yoga to his followers.

These ancient Yogis took the seriousness of the traditional Yoga discipline of their times and integrated it with humor and laughter for the benefit of their students. This humor tradition continues in many of today's contemporary Yoga classes where the practicing mantra is "To laugh is to celebrate and to celebrate is to enjoy the great gift of life itself."

This book was written to share the laughter and joy of the Yoga experience with the millions of Yoga students and teachers worldwide.

We invite you to laugh with us on this light-hearted journey.

Laurence Berkley
Los Angeles, California

CHECK OUT ALL THE LAUGHS AT
YOGALAFFS.COM

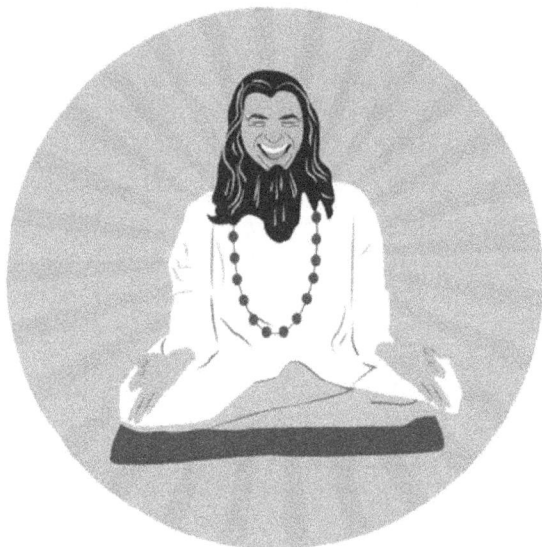

- Special Yoga Laffs Gift Book Orders
- Comedy Yoga Laffs Prints & Art
- Funny Yoga Laffs Tee Shirts
- And Many More Special Offers

All the Funny Yoga Laffs Products in One Great Website... YOGALAFFS.COM

Published by

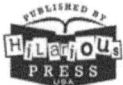

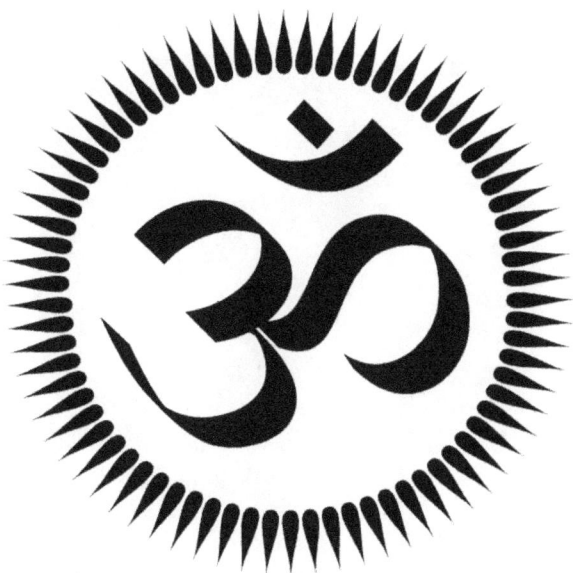

OM
LET THE LAUGHTER
BEGIN...

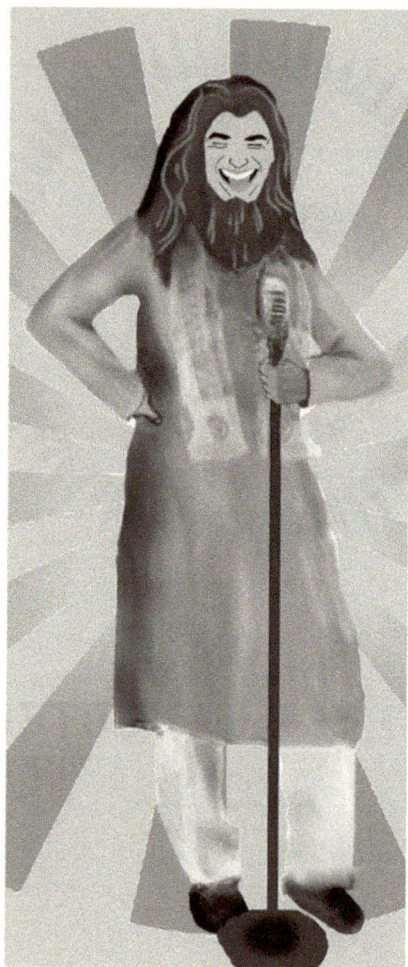

X

Chapter One

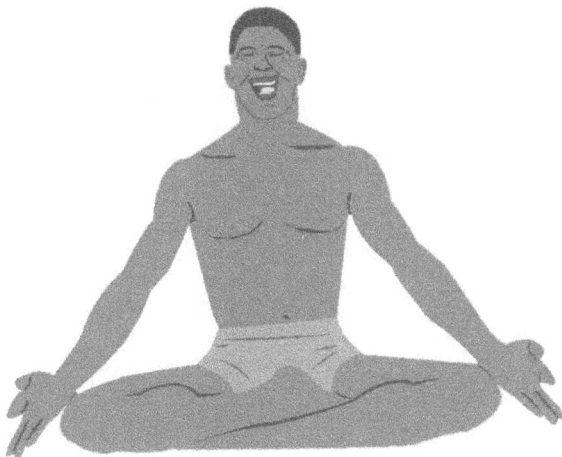

SIDDH ASANA
"Lotus Adapt Pose"

"Blessed are those who are flexible, for they shall never be bent out of shape. Yoga exists in the world because everything is linked."

<u>DESIKASHAR</u>

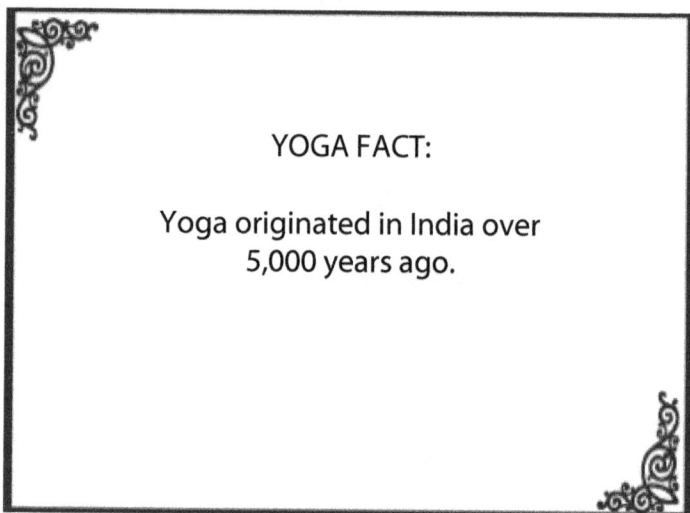

YOGA FACT:

Yoga originated in India over
5,000 years ago.

THERE'S NO PREJUDICE
AT MY ASHRAM.

MY YOGA INSTRUCTOR
TAKES ALL DENOMINATIONS...

10s, 20s, 50s...

According to recent scientific studies from India:

The human race is faced with a cruel choice...

The yoga head stand or daytime television.

KUNDALINI YOGI
SHARPSHOOTER SAYS:

"READY,

AIM,

FIRE!"

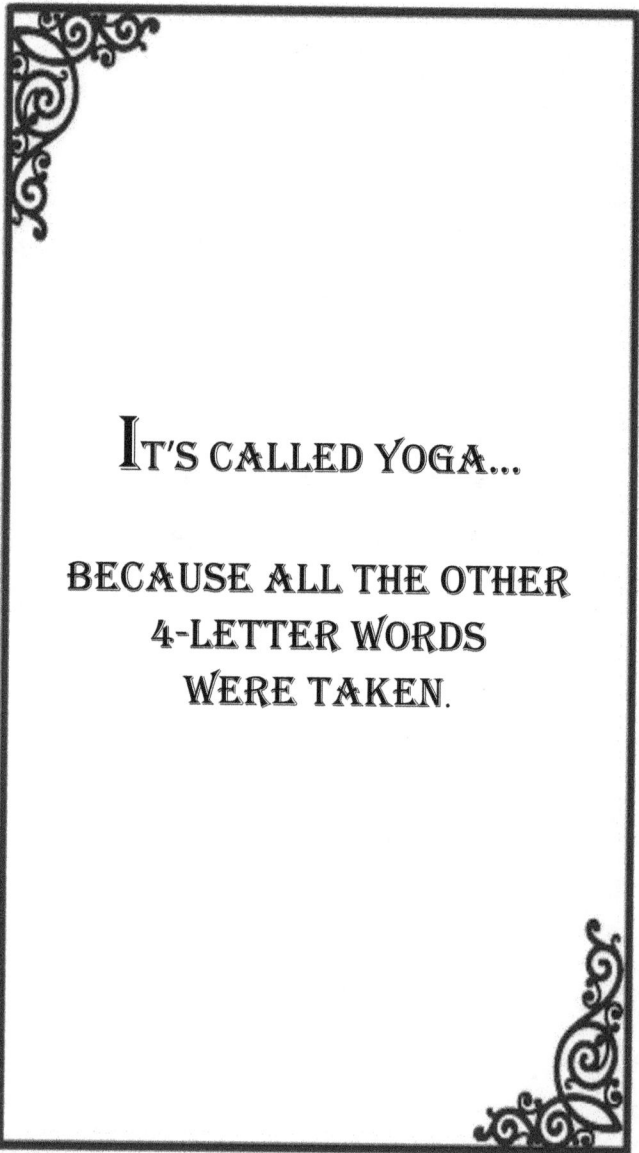

It's called yoga...

Because all the other 4-letter words were taken.

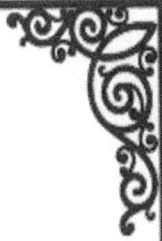

Ashram Class Mantra:

Just don't sit there...
Stretch something!

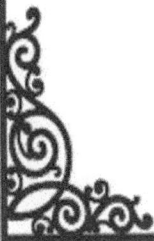

Two Yoga Monks greet
each other in
a Tibetan Ashram...

FIRST MONK: "HOW'S LIFE?"

SECOND MONK: "I'VE HAD
BETTER ONES."

Yogini Training Demands:

DISCIPLINE,
SKILL,
ATHLETICISM AND
PERSEVERANCE...

AND THAT'S JUST TO GET
INTO YOUR TIGHTS.

A SWAMI IS TALKING
TO HIS YOGA PUPIL...

SWAMI: "DO YOU
UNDERSTAND THAT YOU DON'T
REALLY EXIST?"

PUPIL: "TO WHOM ARE YOU
SPEAKING?"

A LOS ANGELES YOGA
STUDENT SPEAKS:

AFTER 12 YEARS OF COSTLY

PERSONAL YOGA TRAINING,
OUTRAGEOUS CLASS FEES,
EXPENSIVE CLOTHING,

AND PRICEY ACCESSORIES...

I AM NOW HAVING AN
OUT OF MONEY EXPERIENCE.

A YOGA STUDENT
ASKS THE GURU…

STUDENT: "MASTER, IS IT
PROPER FOR A MONK TO
USE E-MAIL?"

GURU: "YES, AS LONG AS
THERE ARE NO
ATTACHMENTS."

A TIRED, 30-YEAR YOGA STUDENT SPEAKS:

"WHEN I DIE, I'D LIKE TO COME BACK TO EARTH AS AN OYSTER...

THEN, I'D ONLY HAVE TO DO YOGA FROM SEPTEMBER TO APRIL."

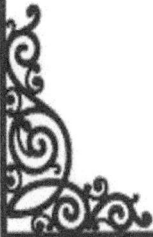

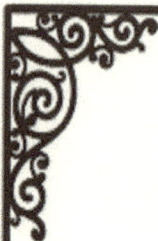

I HAD TO QUIT MY
YOGA TRAINING...

I REALLY WANTED TO
HAVE A GOOD BODY...

BUT NOT AS MUCH AS I
WANTED DESSERT.

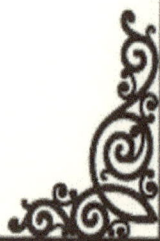

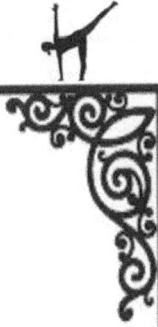

My wife and I are into holistic yoga...

We both wanted natural childbirth...

So, we had our baby on a bed of lettuce in the Whole Foods Market's produce section.

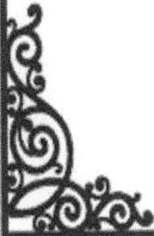

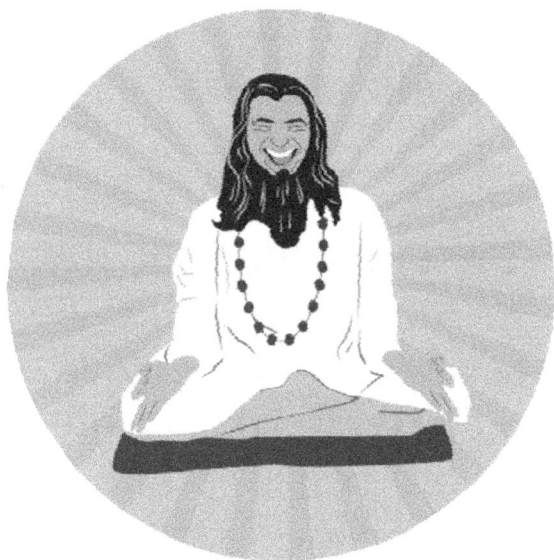

Chapter Two

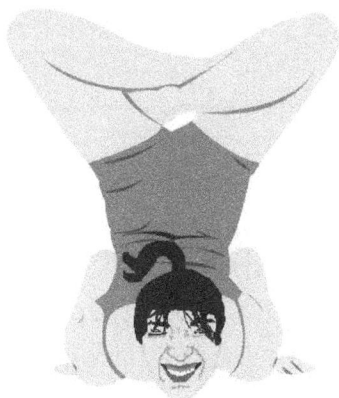

PADMA VIPARITA SALABH ASANA
"Locust Pose"

"Before you've practiced, the theory is useless. After you've practiced, the theory is obvious."
DAVID WILLIAMS, ASHTANGA TEACHER

YOGA FACT:

It is believed that there are more people
practicing Yoga in California than
in all of India.

EVERYBODY IS DOING
YOGA THESE DAYS.

BUT NOT ME...

IF I WANTED TO STAND ON
MY HANDS WITH MY LEGS
BEHIND MY HEAD,
I'D JOIN THE CIRCUS.

Q. Why did the hot yoga instructor cross the road?

A. Because some of his students on the other side could still move.

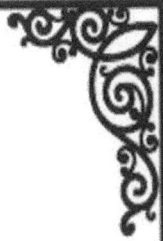

An overweight yoga student speaks:

The toughest part of ashram training for me

Is getting on & off the yoga mat.

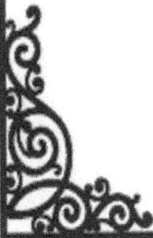

I PREFER YOGA SIT-UPS
TO THE ONE-LEGGED
TREE POSE.

AT LEAST WITH THE YOGA
SIT-UP, I GET TO LIE DOWN
AFTER EACH ONE.

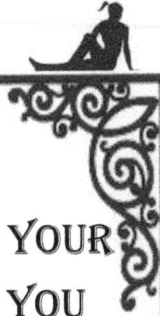

Before you start your ashram training, you must decide whether to take an Ashtanga yoga or an Iyengar yoga program.

It is a difficult choice that all yoga students have to make.

It's not a great choice...

It's sort of like when the doctor says, "Ointment or suppository?"

Two yoga gurus pass
on a mountain
road in Tibet...

First guru says "Hello."

The second guru thinks for
a moment and says to
himself: "I wonder what he
meant by that?

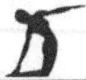

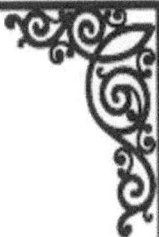

I DECIDED TO JOIN A
REINCARNATION CLUB AT MY
ASHRAM. BUT THEY SAID
MEMBERSHIP WAS $750.

I THOUGHT THAT WAS
PRETTY EXPENSIVE.

BUT THEN I THOUGHT,
"WHAT THE HELL? YOU
ONLY LIVE TWICE."

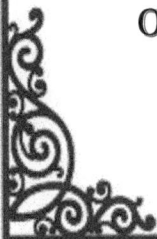

Yoga classes turned
my life around!

I used to be miserable
and depressed...

And now I'm depressed
and miserable.

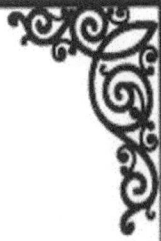

My yoga training program doesn't have to make sense...

I'm the yoga teacher.

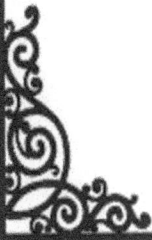

A LADY WAS SPEEDING IN HER NEW CAR AS SHE DROVE TO HER DAILY YOGA CLASS WHEN A COP STOPPED HER AND ASKED:

<u>COP</u>: "WHERE DO YOU THINK YOU'RE GOING IN SUCH A HURRY?"

<u>LADY</u>: "I'M SORRY OFFICER, BUT I'M REALLY SICK."

THE COP LOOKS INTO CAR AND SEES ALL KINDS OF YOGA PARAPHERNALIA AND GEAR.

<u>COP</u>: "SICK? IT LOOKS LIKE YOU'RE GOING TO YOUR YOGA CLASS."

<u>LADY</u>: "OFFICER, DON'T YOU THINK THAT IS A SICKNESS?"

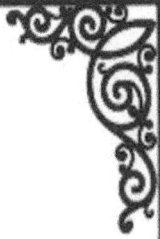

I PRACTICE MY YOGA 7 DAYS A WEEK.

I AM MOTIVATED.
I AM INVINCIBLE.
I AM TIRED.

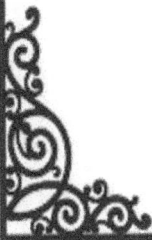

I LOVE MY YOGA CLASS
I LOVE MY YOGA EXERCISES
I LOVE MY YOGA TEACHER
I LOVE MY NEW MEDICATIONS.

I HAD TO GO ON
TWO YOGA DIETS...

ONE DIDN'T GIVE ME
ENOUGH TO EAT.

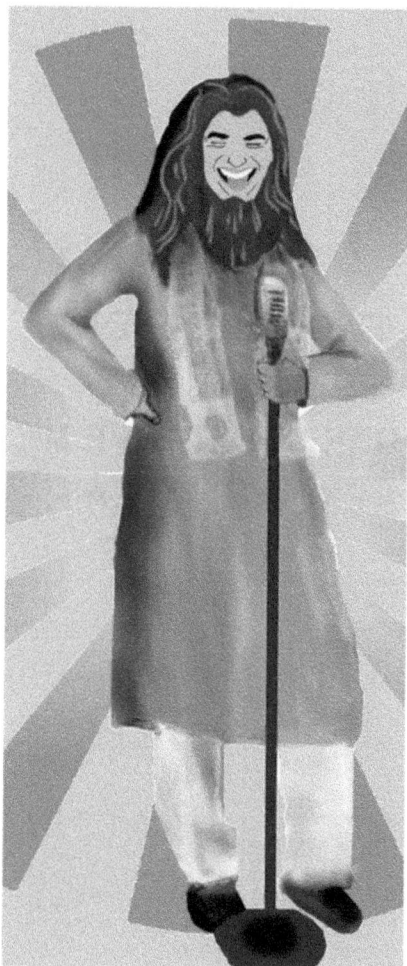

Chapter Three

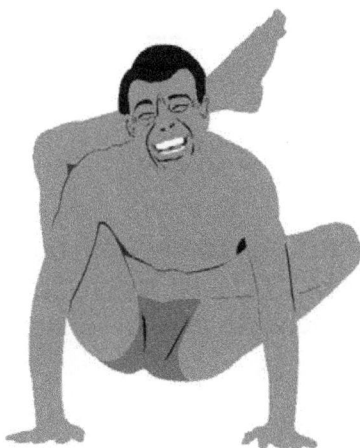

VIRANCHY ASANA
"Dedicated Pose"

"Yoga teaches us to cure that which need not be endured and endure what cannot be endured."

BKS IYENGAR

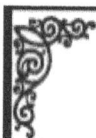

YOGA FACT:

The word Yoga comes from the Sanskrit word "yoke." It can be loosely translated to mean "to join" or "unite."

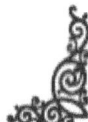

I DON'T NEED YOGA
TRAINING; I HAVE
THE BODY OF A GOD...

UNFORTUNATELY,
IT'S BUDDHA.

The Ashram Student Asks:

Does Running Late to Class Count as a Yoga Exercise?

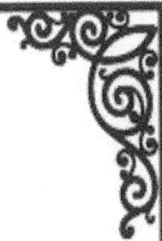

<u>AN EX YOGA STUDENT SPEAKS:</u>

Yoga class workouts
fascinate me...

I could sit and watch
them for hours.

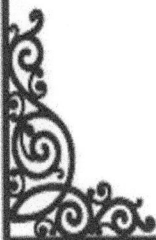

A YOGINI SPEAKS:

YOGA WOMEN DON'T HAVE HOT FLASHES.

WE HAVE POWER SURGES.

Yoga t-shirt:

I'm a yoga student.
This is as happy as i get.

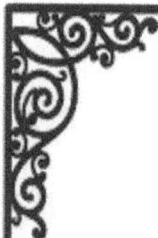

Yoga was never for me...

My idea of a balanced diet is a glazed doughnut in each hand.

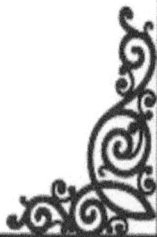

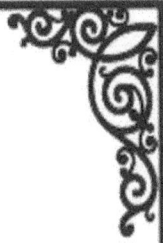

Ashram Studio Rules:

Rule #1:
The Yoga Teacher is always right.

Rule #2:
If the Yoga Teacher's wrong, see Rule #1.

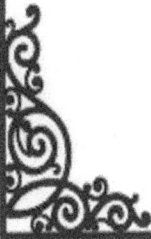

I AM NOT AN OBSESSIVE YOGINI
I AM NOT AN OBSESSIVE YOGINI
I AM NOT AN OBSESSIVE YOGINI
I AM NOT AN OBSESSIVE YOGINI
I AM NOT AN OBSESSIVE YOGINI

A NEW YOGA STUDENT SPEAKS:

I BELIEVE IN MIRACLES...

I HAVE TO...

THEY'RE A MAJOR PART OF MY YOGA WEIGHT LOSS PROGRAM.

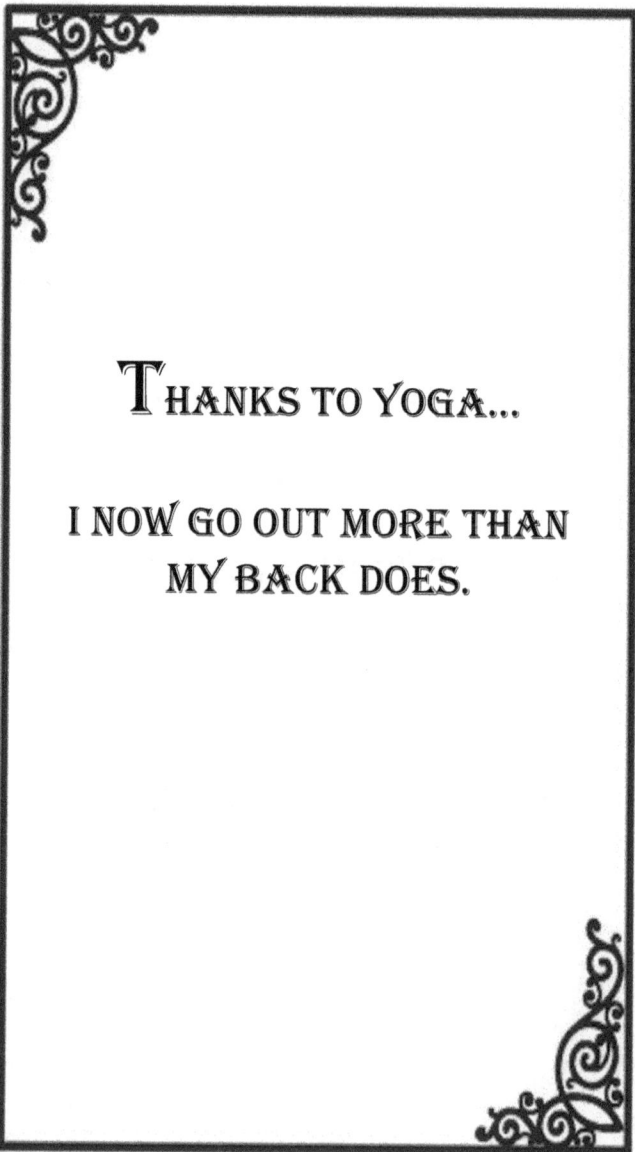

Thanks to yoga...

I now go out more than
my back does.

Wisdsom of the Maharishi:

Change is inevitable...

Except from a vending machine.

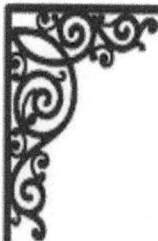

Consciousness...

THAT ANNOYING TIME BETWEEN YOGA CLASSES.

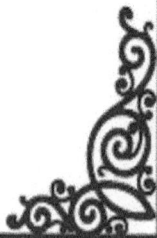

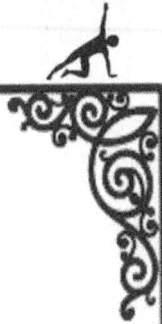

THE PUPIL ASKS
THE MAHARISHI:

IF A YOGI SHOUTS OUT HIS
FEELINGS IN THE
FOREST AND THERE IS
NO YOGINI AROUND
TO HEAR HIM...

IS HE STILL WRONG?

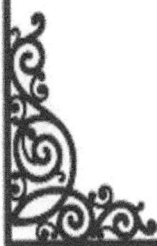

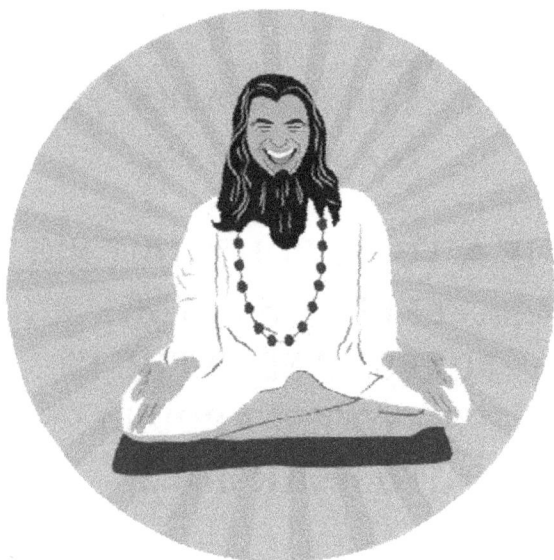

CHAPTER 4

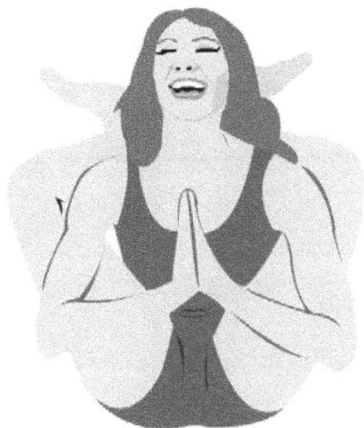

DWI PADA SIRS ASANA
"Behind Head Pose"

"A photographer gets people to pose for him. A Yoga instructor gets people to pose for themselves."

<u>T. GUILLEMETS</u>

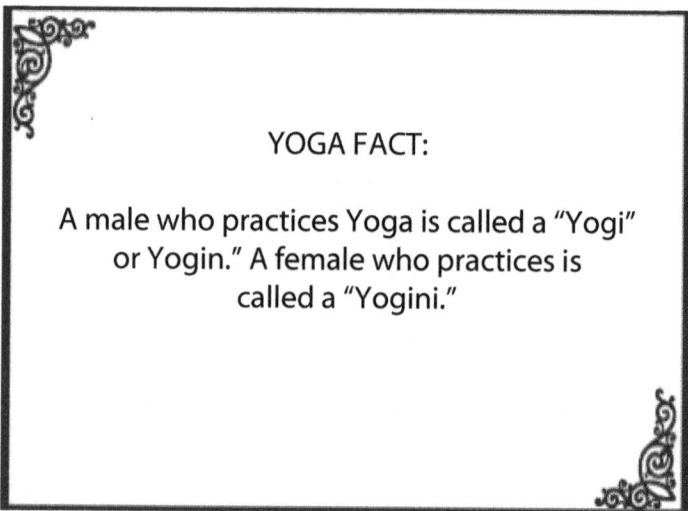

YOGA FACT:

A male who practices Yoga is called a "Yogi" or Yogin." A female who practices is called a "Yogini."

In some cultures,
what I do in my yoga class
would be considered
normal.

I WAS EXCITED AFTER
MY FIRST THREE
YOGA CLASSES...

I TOLD MY TEACHER THAT
I WANTED TO DO
YOGA VERY BADLY.

SHE SAID I SUCCEEDED.

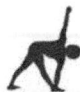

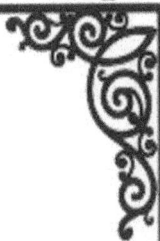

It may look like I'm doing nothing physical in my yoga class...

But on a cellular level, I'm really quite busy.

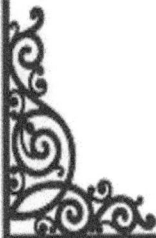

WISDOM OF THE MAHARISHI:

SEX IS ONE OF THE NINE REASONS FOR REINCARNATION.

THE OTHER EIGHT ARE UNIMPORTANT.

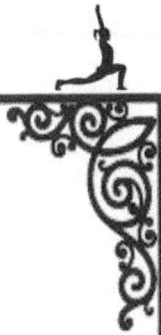

Yoga student's mantra:

I BEND
SO I DON'T BREAK.

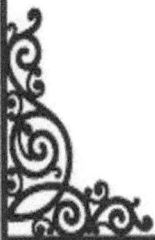

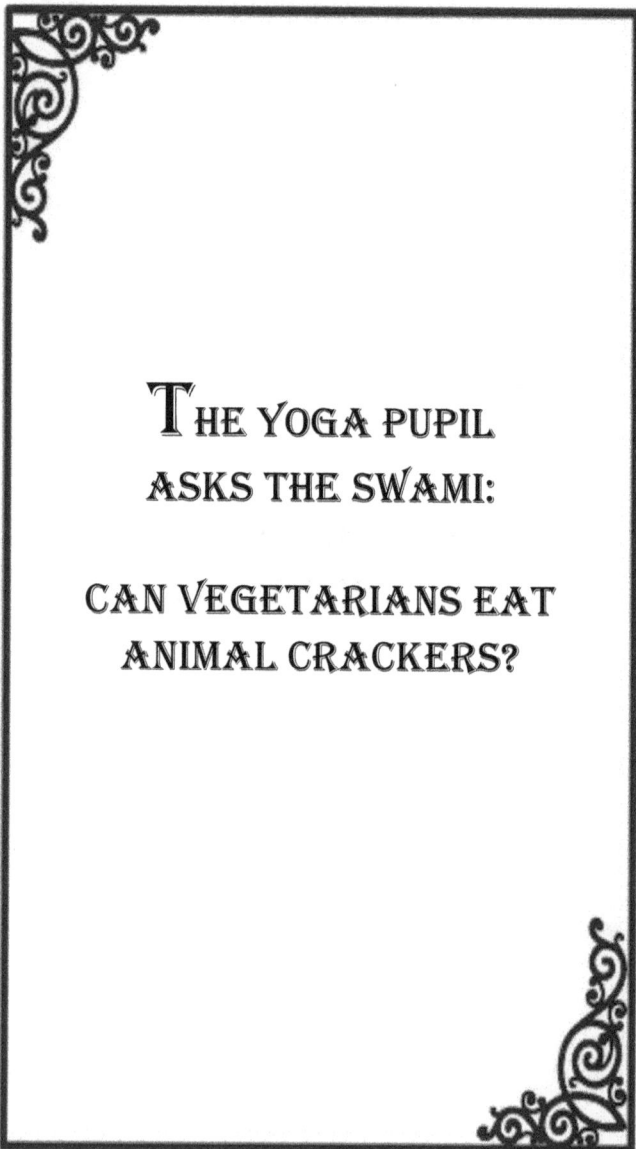

THE YOGA PUPIL ASKS THE SWAMI:

CAN VEGETARIANS EAT ANIMAL CRACKERS?

Wisdom of the swami:

A yogini has the last word in any argument.

Anything a yogi says after that, is the beginning of a new argument.

Wisdom of the maharishi:

If you die in an elevator,
make sure you
press the up button.

Ex Yoga Student Speaks:

Yoga Training Allowed Me To Say No To Drugs And Alcohol...

But They Just Didn't Listen!

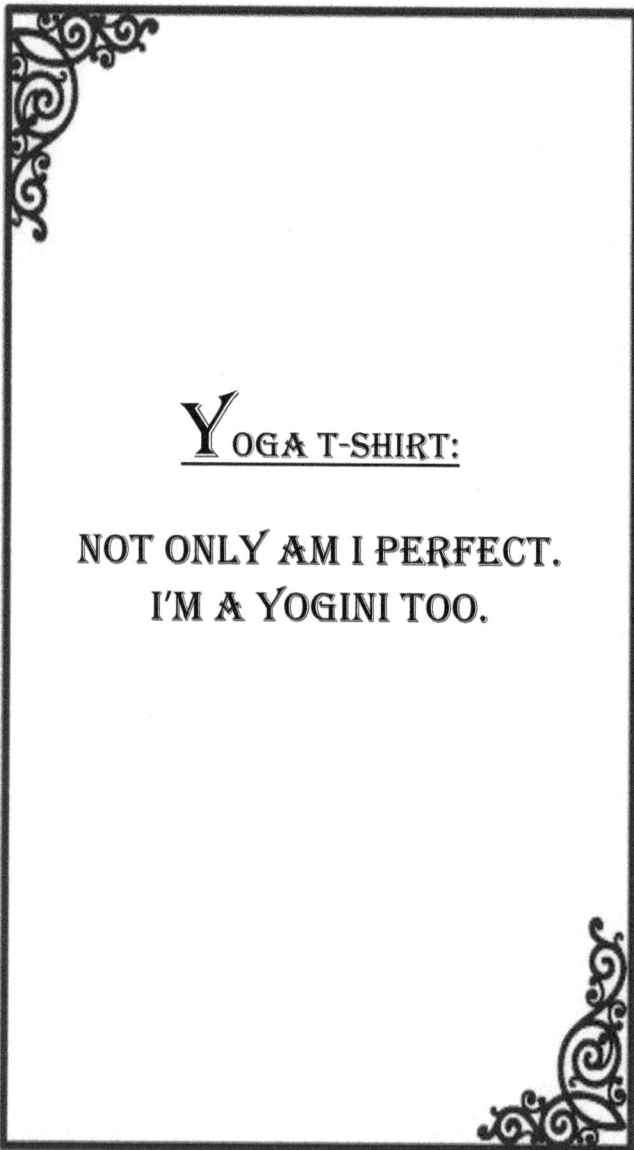

Yoga t-shirt:

Not only am I perfect. I'm a Yogini too.

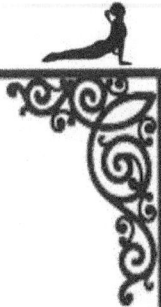

Q: **W**HAT DID THE YOGA GURU SAY TO THE HOTDOG VENDOR?

A: "MAKE ME ONE WITH EVERYTHING."

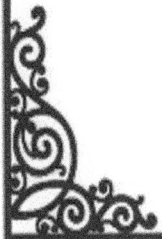

Wisdom of the maharishi:

Live every day
as if it was your last...

And then one day
you'll be right.

THE YOGA PUPIL ASKS THE MAHARISHI:

IF BEAUTY IS TRUTH...

THEN WHY DON'T YOGINIS GO TO THE COURTHOUSE TO GET THEIR HAIR DONE?

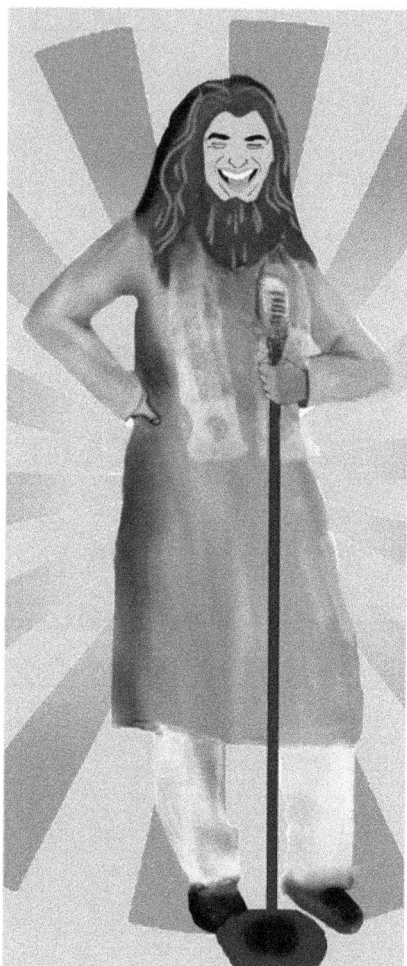

CHAPTER 5

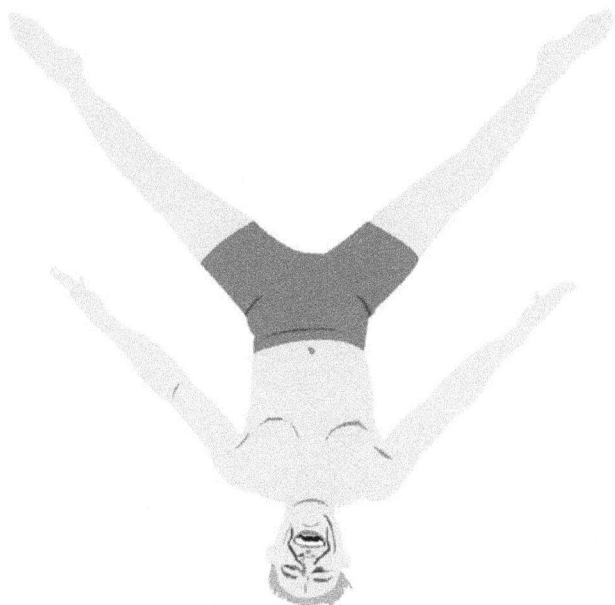

NIRALAMBA SIRSANA
"Unsupported Head Pose"

"The calm steadiness of the senses is called Yoga. Then one should become watchful, because Yoga comes and goes."
KATHA UPANISHAD

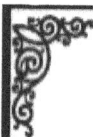

YOGA FACT:

Hatha Yoga is the type of Yoga that transforms exercise and is the form that most people are familiar with.

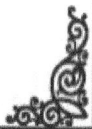

Vegetarian:

A Native American word meaning "lousy hunter"

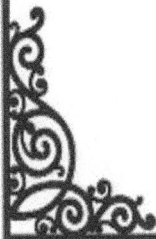

<u>A NEW YOGA STUDENT SPEAKS:</u>

I AM NOT LAZY WHEN IT
COMES TO DOING MY
ASANAS IN CLASS...

I'M JUST MOTIVATIONALLY
CHALLENEGED.

THE MAHARISHI SAYS:

"FOLLOW YOUR DREAMS...

EXCEPT FOR ONE WHERE
YOU'RE NAKED IN YOUR
YOGA CLASS."

Ashram Wall Grafitti:

SAVE THE EARTH!

IT'S OUR ONLY SOURCE OF CHOCOLATE!

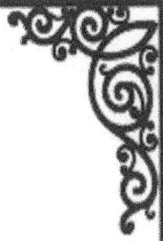

IN YOGA TRAINING,

GETTING ON YOUR FEET,
MEANS GETTING OFF
YOUR BUTT.

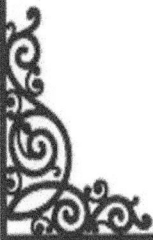

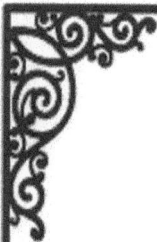

A LOS ANGELES YOGA TEACHER SAYS TO THE NEW HATHA STUDENT:

"THAT'S NOT A YOGA OUTFIT YOU'RE WEARING...

IT'S A CRY FOR HELP."

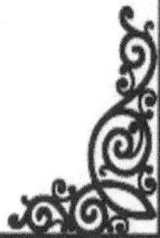

BEING ON TIME FOR MY YOGA CLASS MEANS...

"WHEN I GET THERE."

Ashram Wall Grafitti:

"Vini, Vidi, Visa...

I came,
I saw,
I did a little shopping."

I'M SORRY,
THERE'S ONLY
SO MUCH I CAN DO
FOR YOUR BODY...

I'M A YOGA INSTRUCTOR,
NOT A MAGICIAN.

Q. What has 18 arms, 18 legs and one tooth?

A. A 9 women Yoga class in Arkansas.

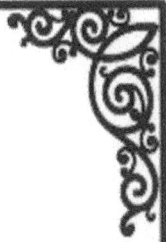

After 5 years
of intensive
ashram training...

The only yoga stretch
I've perfected is
the yawn.

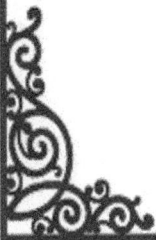

THANKS TO MY
YOGA TEACHINGS,
I THINK I CAN LIVE FOREVER...

SO FAR, SO GOOD

Yoga police:

"You have the right to remain silent!"

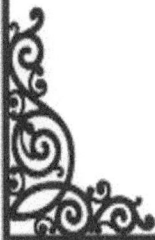

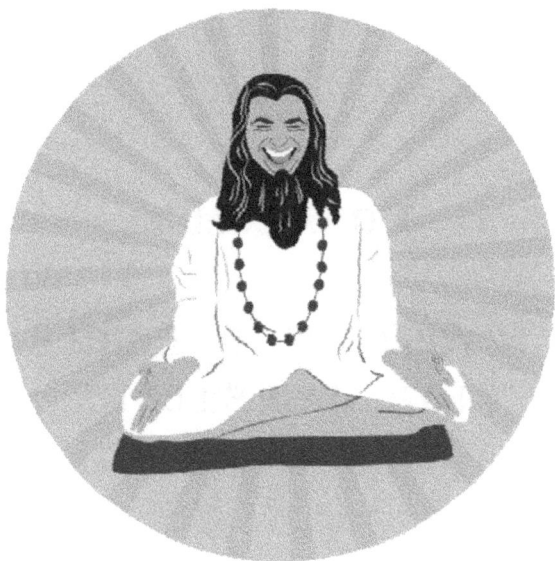

CHAPTER 6

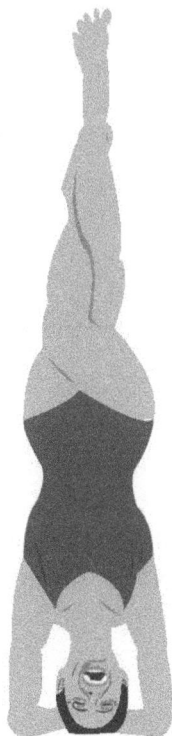

GARUD ASANA INSIRS ASANA
"Headstand With Eagle Legs Pose"

"Yoga is the perfect opportunity to be curious about who you are."

JASON CRANDELL

YOGA FACT:

Over 30 million people do Yoga in
North America.

Q. **W**HY DID THE YOGA MASTER REFUSE NOVOCAINE AT THE DENTIST'S OFFICE?

A. BECAUSE HE WANTED TO TRANSCEND DENTAL MEDICATION.

Ashram Wall Grafitti:

"Vini, Vidi, Velcro...

I came,
I saw,
I stuck around."

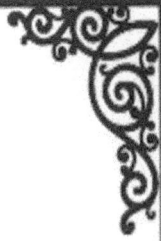

I NAMED MY DOG "KARMA."

"GOOD KARMA!"

"BAD KARMA!!!"

HE'S MUCH EASIER
TO CONTROL NOW.

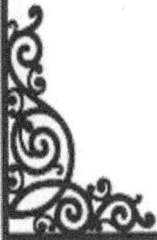

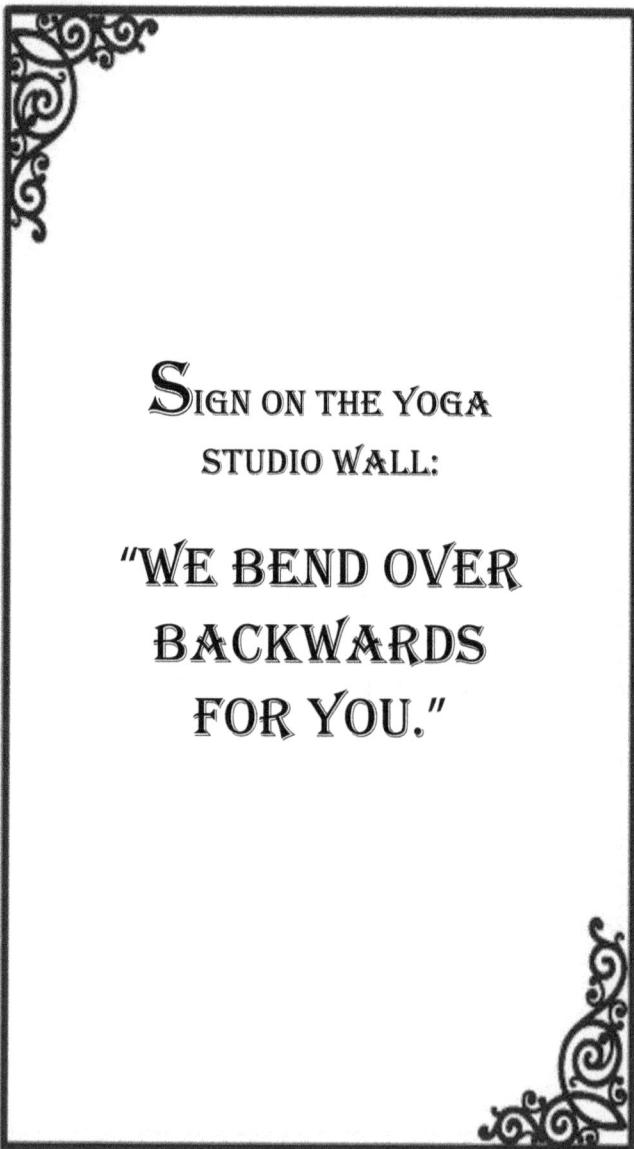

Sign on the yoga
studio wall:

"We bend over backwards for you."

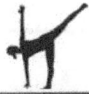
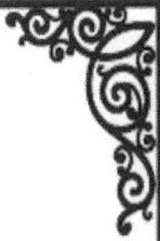

Q. **W**HAT DOES A DYSLEXIC
YOGA COW SAY?

A. "OOOOMMMM."

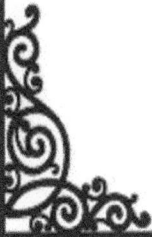

I GIVE A 100% OF MY ENERGY
TO MY DAILY YOGA WORKOUTS:

12% ON MONDAY
23% ON TUESDAY
40% ON WEDNESDAY
20% ON THURSDAY
5% ON FRIDAY

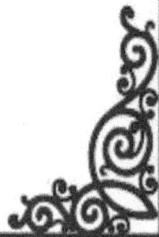

The maharishi proclaims:

I DREAM OF A BETTER WORLD
WHERE CHICKENS CAN CROSS
THE ROAD WITHOUT THEIR
MOTIVES BEING QUESTIONED

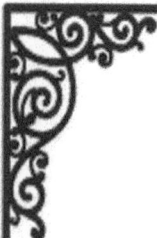

If it weren't for all the
pain, cramps, sprains,
muscle tears,
and fractures...

Hot Yoga would have
the lowest injury
rate of any sports
training program.

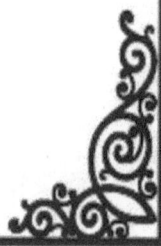

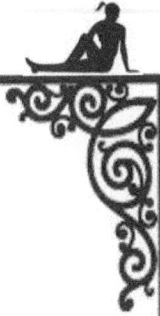

Two men meet on the street...

FIRST MAN: "AND HOW'S YOUR SON? IS HE STILL UNEMPLOYED?"

SECOND MAN: "YES, HE IS. BUT HE IS DOING YOGA MEDITATION NOW."

FIRST MAN: "YOGA MEDITATION? WHAT'S THAT?"

SECOND MAN: "I DON'T KNOW. BUT IT'S BETTER THAN HIM JUST SITTING AROUND THE HOUSE DOING NOTHING!"

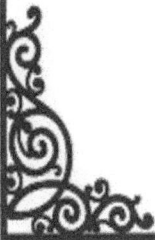

Q. **W**HY COULDN'T THE YOGI OPERATE HIS VACUUM CLEANER?

A. HE'D LOST ALL HIS ATTACHMENTS.

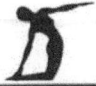

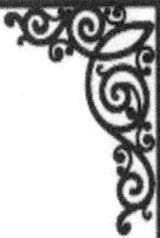

Q. **H**OW MANY HATHA YOGA STUDENTS DOES IT TAKE TO CHANGE A LIGHT BULB?

A. ONE... BUT FIRST THEY'LL HAVE TO DO 5 SUN A'S AND 5 SUN B'S...

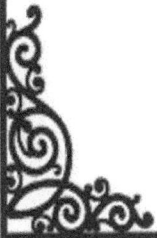

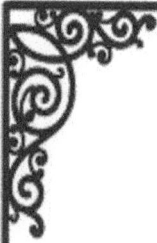

Sign on ashram window:

Yoga instructor wanted.
INQUIRE WITHIN.

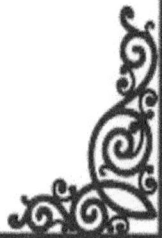

I WOULD DO MORE YOGA
EXERCISES AT HOME...

BUT IT MAKES ME
SPILL MY BEER.

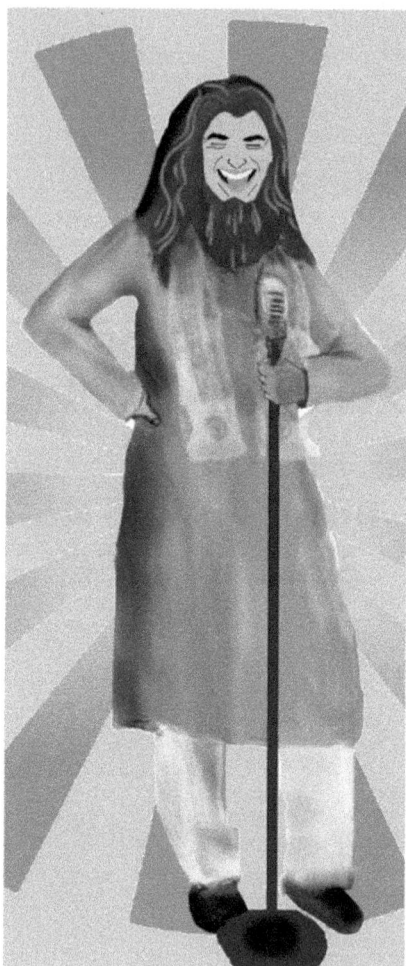

CHAPTER 7

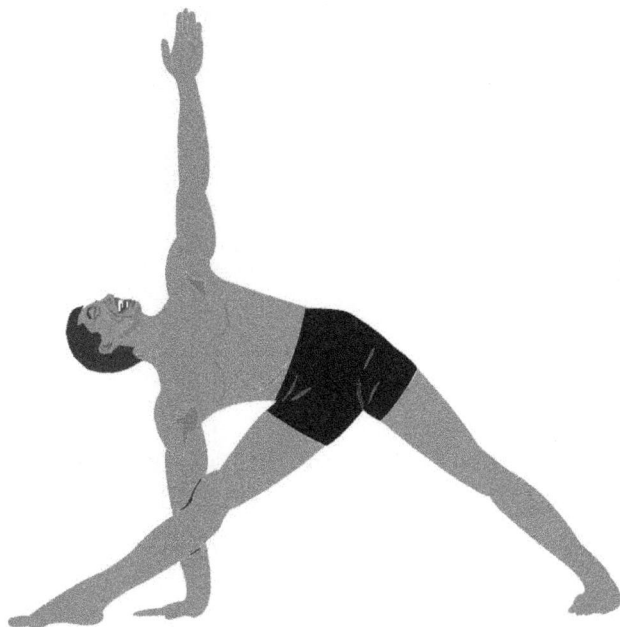

UTTHITATRIKON ASANA
"Extended Triangle Pose"

"The Yoga Mat is a good place to turn to when talk therapy and antidepressants aren't enough."

AMY WEINTRAUB

YOGA FACT:

Yoga can be literally done anywhere.
Variations can be done at your desk, in your
car, or even on an airplane.

Q: **How many tibetan yogis does it take to change a lightbulb?**

A: INTO WHAT?

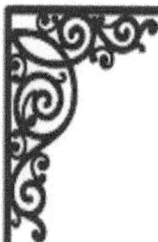

Thanks to yoga,
I never complain
about life...

I merely think of all the
lifetime guarantees I've
outlived.

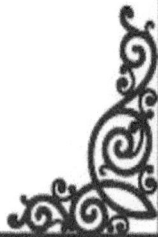

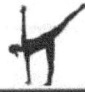

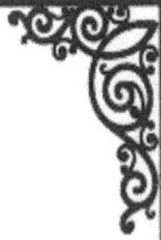

I STARTED OUT WITH
A LOT OF DOUBTS ABOUT
THE BENEFITS OF
YOGA CLASSES…

AND AFTER 3 YEARS
OF TRAINING,
I STILL HAVE
MOST OF THEM LEFT

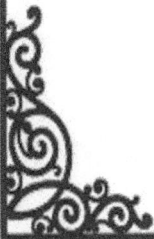

A YOGINI PROCLAIMS:

SINCE TAKING YOGA, I NOW
HAVE A NICE FIGURE.

BEFORE YOGA, MY T-SHIRT
USED TO SAY:

"BODY BY BEN & JERRY'S."

After a particularly 'snobbish' student did a really bad solo performance of various asanas for her hatha class, she arrogantly walks over to the instructor and asks:

STUDENT: "What did you think of my execution?"

INSTRUCTOR: "I'm all in favor of it."

Ashram wall graffiti:

DOGMA IS MAN'S BEST FRIEND!

A PARTICULARLY IRRITATING AND EGOTISTICAL YOGA STUDENT WAS CHATTING WITH HER TEACHER.

STUDENT: "HOW MANY TRULY GREAT YOGA STUDENTS HAVE YOU TAUGHT?"

TEACHER: "ONE LESS THAN YOU THINK."

Sign on the ashram wall:

YOGA TRAINING
TAKES ITS TOLL...

PLEASE HAVE
EXACT CHANGE.

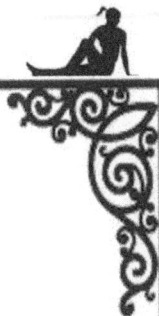

BEFORE YOGA, MY
NUTRITIONAL KNOWLEDGE
WAS SO BAD, I USED TO
THINK THE 4 BASIC
FOOD GROUPS WERE:

1. FAST;
2. JUNK;
3. FROZEN;
4. BROWN BAG.

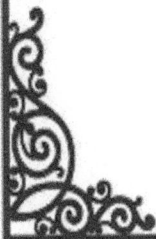

Homeless yoga student carrying a sign in front of the ashram:

"I WILL DO ASANAS FOR FOOD!"

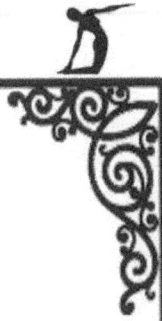

I WAS GOING TO DO
SOMETHING NICE FOR MY
YOGA TEACHER...

BUT I DIDN'T WANT TO
SET A PRECEDENT.

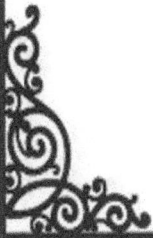

On a TV interview show, the celebrity yoga instructor said to the host:

CELEBRITY: "It took me 25 years to realize that I know nothing about yoga."

HOST: "Then why didn't you quit?"

CELEBRITY: It was too late to quit. By that time, I had already become a yoga authority."

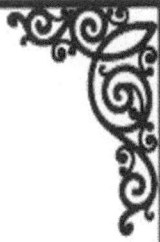

AN EX YOGA STUDENT SPEAKS:

I WAS THROWN OUT OF COLLEGE FOR CHEATING ON MY METAPHYSICS EXAM.

I WAS CAUGHT LOOKING INTO THE SOUL OF THE BOY SITTING NEXT TO ME.

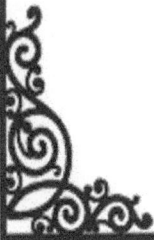

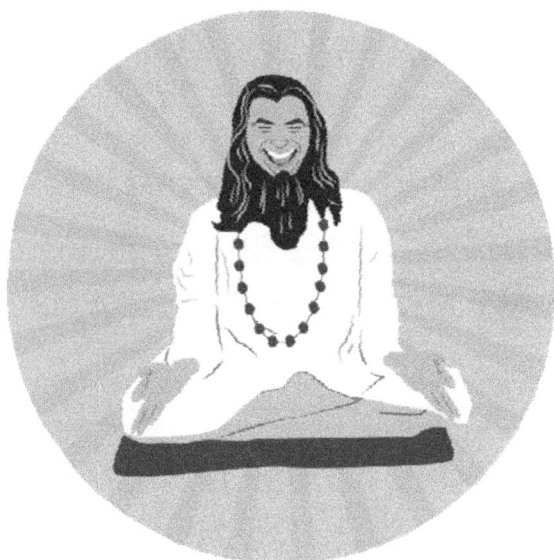

CHAPTER 8

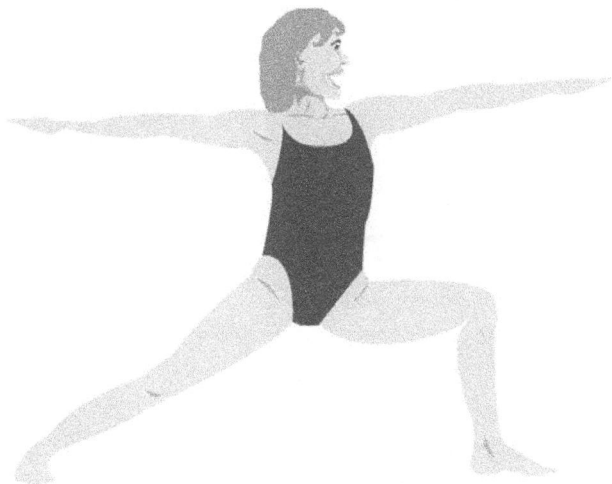

VIRAVHADR ASANA
"Warrior Pose"

"Yoga is the fountain of youth. You're only as young as your spine is flexible."
BOB HARPER

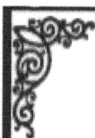

YOGA FACT:

Everyone can do Yoga. Asanas can be
modified to accommodate
any physical limitations.

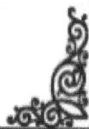

A MEDICAL PROBLEM:

A YOGA INSTRUCTOR WAS SITTING IN THE DOCTOR'S OFFICE AND TELLING THE MEDIC ABOUT HAVING UNBELIEVABLE MUSCLE SPASMS IN WHICH HIS ARMS SHOT STRAIGHT IN TO THE AIR AND HE SHOOK VIOLENTLY.

INSTRUCTOR: "WHAT CAN I DO, DOCTOR?"

DOCTOR: "WELL, MY FIRST ADVICE IS TO STAY AWAY FROM AUCTIONS."

Now, THANKS TO MY
YOGA TRAINING,
I HAVE A BLACK
BELT IN KARATE...

IT'S NOT THAT I'M
GOOD AT IT...

IT'S JUST THAT I
NEVER WASH IT.

Even though my wife
is overweight,
she doesn't have to go to
her yoga classes
anymore...

she gets enough exercise
just trying to get in to
her leotards.

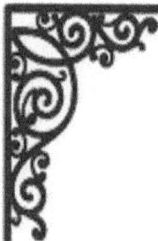

I'M NOT INTO
VIGOROUS YOGA WORKOUTS...

MY EXERCISE MANTRA IS:

"NO PAIN, NO PAIN."

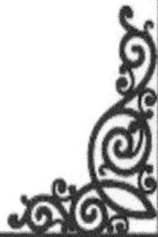

St. paddy's day yoga greeting:

"TOP OF THE MAT TO YA."

Yoga teaches:

THERE'S VERY LITTLE
DIFFERENCE BETWEEN
A VEGETARIAN AND
A MEAT EATER.

VEGETABLES ARE LIVING
THINGS, TOO...

THEY'RE JUST
EASIER TO CATCH.

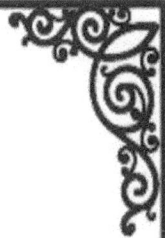

MANY WEALTHY PEOPLE DON'T DO YOGA FOR RELIGIOUS REASONS.

THEY FIGURE, IF GOD HAD WANTED THEM TO BEND OVER...

HE WOULD HAVE PUT CASH ON THE FLOOR.

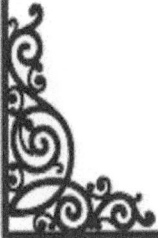

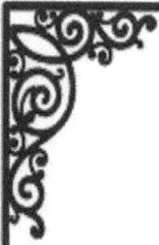

I'M MIDDLE AGED
AND DIVORCED.

THE ONLY REASON I
TOOK UP YOGA IS SO THAT
I COULD HEAR THE SOUND
OF HEAVY BREATHING AGAIN.

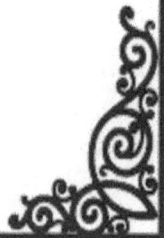

Yoga success story:

THANKS TO MY INTENSIVE
YOGA TRAINING,
I FINISHED THE NEW YORK
CITY MARATHON
IN UNDER AN HOUR...

IT WOULD HAVE BEEN FASTER,
BUT I HAD TO STOP FOR GAS.

I JOINED A YOGA CLASS
LAST YEAR TO LOSE WEIGHT.

I SPENT $700 FOR PERSONAL
ASHRAM TRAINING.
I HAVEN'T LOST A POUND YET.

BUT PEOPLE KEEP
TELLING ME,
"YOU DON'T UNDERSTAND THE
PRINCIPLE HERE...

YOU HAVE TO SHOW
UP TO CLASS."

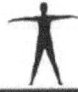

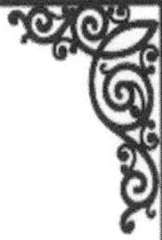

YOGA MEN SAY THEY GET
THEIR BEST EXERCISE
IN THE BEDROOM.

BECAUSE THEY FEEL
THAT'S WHERE
THEY GET THE MOST
RESISTANCE.

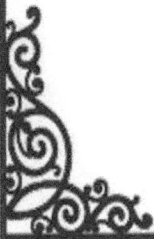

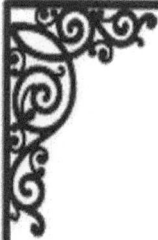

My wife is doing yoga training for travel reasons.

She's trying to stop her tush from going south without her.

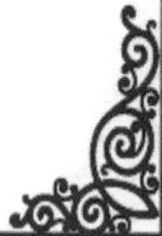

My doctor told me to take yoga to get into shape...

I told him:
"BUT DOC, ROUND IS A SHAPE."

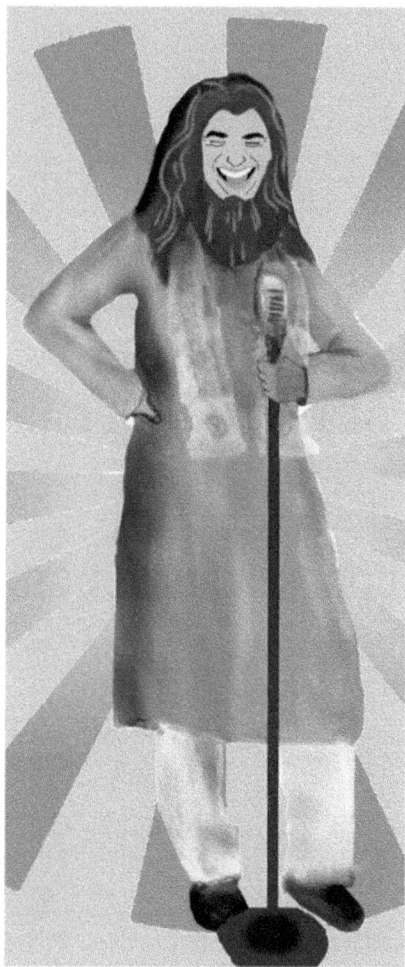

CHAPTER 9

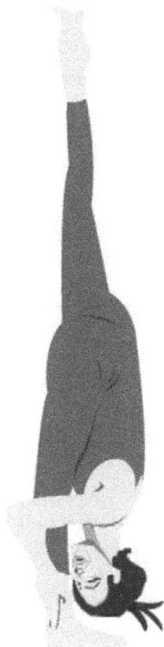

URDHVA PRASARITA EKE PAD ASANA

"One Legged Forward Bend Pose"

"I do Yoga so that I can stay flexible enough to kick my own ass if necessary."
BETSY CANAS GARMON

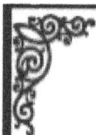

YOGA FACT:

Yoga and diet go hand in hand. There are certain foods you can eat that can actually increase your flexibility and brain function.

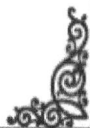

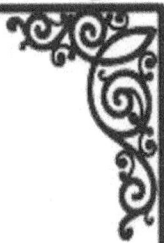

Life's not fair...

As if getting up in the morning isn't bad enough, it has to be followed by your yoga class.

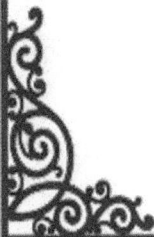

THE MAHARISHI SAYS:

TO PERFECT YOUR
YOGA TRAINING...

WORK LIKE A DOG,
EAT LIKE A HORSE,
THINK LIKE A FOX,
PLAY LIKE A RABBIT...

AND SEE YOUR
VETERINARIAN
TWICE A YEAR.

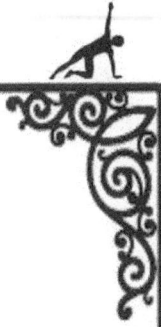

YOGA PHILOSOPHY TEACHES:

TO LIVE TO BE A HUNDRED,
YOU FIRST MUST
GET TO BE 99...

THEN BE VERY CAREFUL FOR
THE NEXT YEAR.

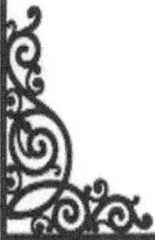

My doctor told me that
yoga could add
years to my life.

He's right.

After 3 months
of yoga training,
I feel 20 years older.

I KNEW I WAS PUTTING ON WEIGHT AND NEEDED TO SIGN UP FOR YOGA CLASSES...

WHEN MY WIFE HAD TO LET OUT THE SHOWER CURTAIN.

Yoga training has been emotionally painful for me.

I told my instructor that in 10 years of being in his class, he's never once said anything nice about my yoga technique.

He asked for a little more time.

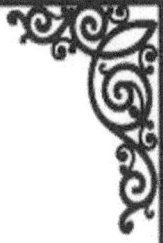

How come you never see a smiling student in a hot yoga class?

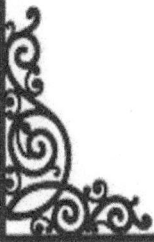

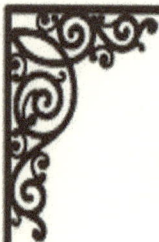

The guru says:

A yoga class melt down is not some kind of a cheese sandwich.

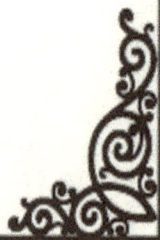

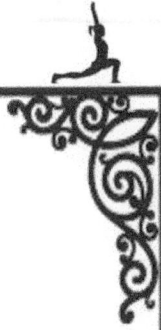

THERE'S ONLY ONE THING
HOLDING ME BACK
FROM PERFECTING
MY YOGA TECHNIQUE...

MY BACK.

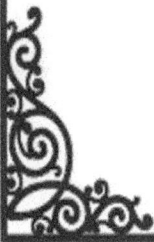

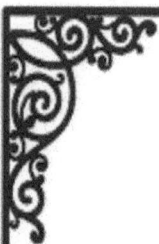

In los angeles, there's a telephone hotline for yoga students in denial...

So far, no one has called.

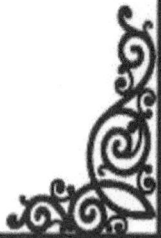

THE MAHARISHI SAYS:

IT'S A SMALL WORLD...

BUT I WOULDN'T WANT
TO PAINT IT.

My teacher is not
the worst yoga
instructor in L.A...

But until a worse
one comes along,
he'll do.

I PHONED OUR LOCAL ASHRAM TO SIGN UP FOR THE YOGA FITNESS PROGRAM.

THE INSTRUCTOR TOLD ME THAT WHEN I ARRIVE AT CLASS, TO MAKE SURE I WEAR LOOSE FITTING CLOTHING...

I SAID: "LOOK, IF I HAD ANY LOOSE-FITTING CLOTHING, I WOULDN'T NEED THE YOGA CLASS."

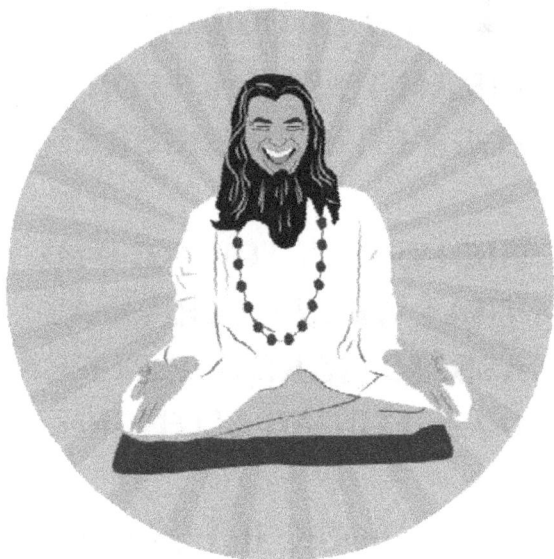

CHAPTER 10

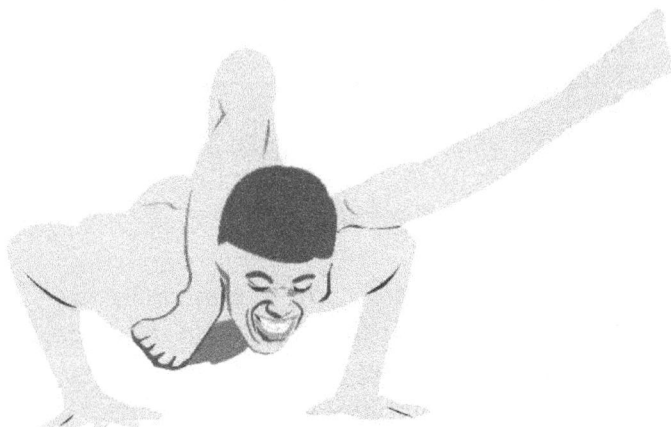

VALGUL ASANA
"Bat Pose"

"You cannot do Yoga. Yoga is your natural state. What you can do are Yoga exercises, which may reveal to you where you are resisting your natural state."

SHARON GANNO

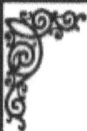

YOGA FACT:

The Sanskrit word "Om" is found in Hindu and Tibetan philosophy. It is said to be the primordial sound of the universe and is connected to the Ajna Chakra (the conscience) or "third eye" region.

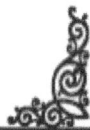

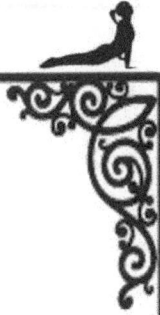

ACCORDING TO SOME YOGA TEACHINGS, IF THERE REALLY WAS SUCH A THING AS REINCARNATION...

THEN HEAVEN WOULD ONLY BE A PLACE TO STOP OFF & PICK UP CLEAN LAUNDRY.

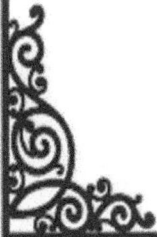

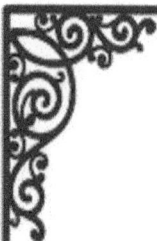

My yoga partner is very flexible.

He is a man with...

His shoulder to the wheel; his nose to the grindstone; his ear to the ground...

The worst yoga posture I've ever seen.

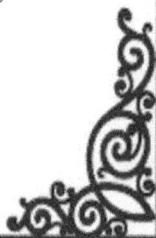

My mother is very religious.

She said we were all born to suffer...

So I married a yoga student

I HAD TO QUIT MY YOGA
CLASS BECAUSE
I BROKE A TOE...

UNFORTUNATELY, IT WAS
MY TEACHER'S.

When asked what gifts he wanted for his birthday, the guru replied:

"I wish for no gifts, only presence."

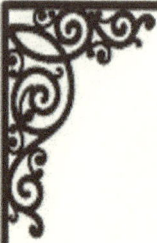

Yoga instructor says to late arriving student:

"You should have been here at nine o'clock."

The student replies: "Why, what happened then?"

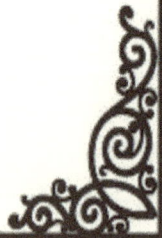

Even though my wife and i
are getting a divorce...

We still do yoga
meditation together.

She is an earth sign and
i'm a water sign.

Together we make mud.

A SENIOR YOGA STUDENT SPEAKS:

"I PERSONALLY DON'T MIND
GROWING OLD...

BUT MY BODY'S
TAKING IT BADLY."

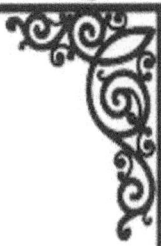

Wisdom of the Maharishi:

Don't judge someone until you have walked a mile in their shoes...

Then they are a mile away and you have their shoes.

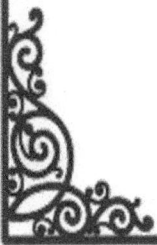

Q. **W**HY DID THE ARTHRITIC YOGI MAKE A CLAIM FOR DISABILITY BENEFITS?

A. BECAUSE HE COULD NO LONGER MAKE ENDS MEET.

SOME PEOPLE CLAIM TO
ENJOY YOGA TRAINING...

BUT, THEN AGAIN, SOME
PEOPLE CLAIM TO HAVE BEEN
ABDUCTED BY ALIENS, TOO.

Ex yoga student speaks:

I never thought I'd be the type to get up early in the morning to do my yoga exercises...

And I was right.

I KNEW THAT MY YOGA TEACHER NEVER LIKED ME.

HE CONSTANTLY COMPLAINED ABOUT MY ATTENDANCE PROBLEM...

I WAS ALWAYS PRESENT.

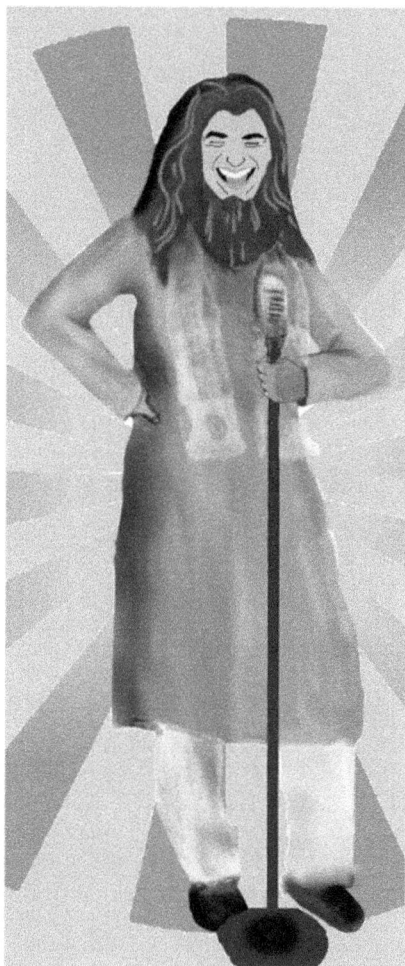

CHAPTER 11

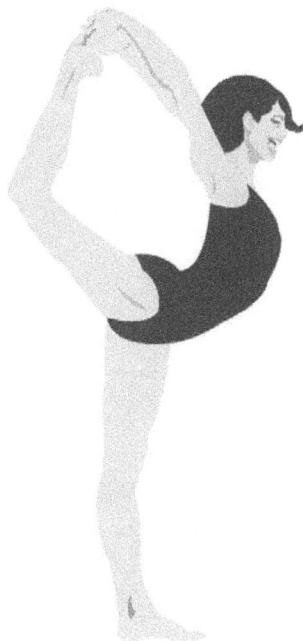

NATARA ASANA
"Dance Pose"

"When the breath wanders, the mind also is
unsteady. But when the breath is calmed, the mind,
too, will be still, and the Yogi achieves long life.
Therefore, one should learn to control the breath."
HATHA YOGA PRADIPIKA

YOGA FACT:

Several scholars have noted that Yoga had been packaged so well as a defense against illness and aging that it is "easy to lose sight of its real purpose—spiritual liberation."

Q. **W**HAT DID THE TIBETAN YOGI SAY TO THE TIBETAN YOGINI AFTER SEX?

A. "THAT WAS WONDERFUL FOR YOU.

HOW WAS IT FOR ME?"

Wisdom of the Maharishi:

Never go mountain climbing with a beneficiary.

I'M NOT DOING TOO WELL WITH
MY MEDITATION TRAINING.

IT'S TRUE, THAT I AM
CONNECTED WITH
MY YOGA REALITY...

BUT, UNFORTUNATELY,
IT'S A BAD CONNECTION.

My yoga exercise class
is a fairy tale...

GRIMM.

Before i started yoga, there was only one thing harder than my muscles…

My arteries.

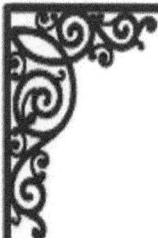

Warning sign in a
hatha Yoga class:

Caution:
Slow moving seniors

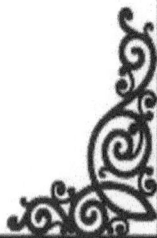

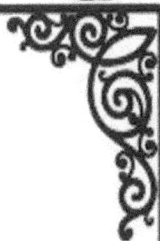

YOGA IS AN ANCIENT
SANSKRIT WORD
THAT MEANS:

"HEAL YOUR BODY...

WITHOUT HEALTH INSURANCE."

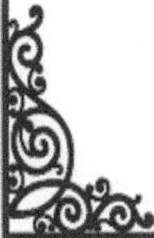

Yoga philosophy:

The age of thirty-five is when you finally get your head together...

And your body starts falling apart.

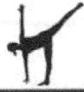

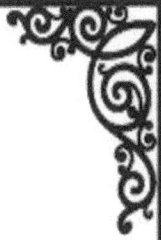

I HATE IT WHEN MY FOOT FALLS ASLEEP DURING YOGA CLASS...

BECAUSE THAT MEANS IT'S GOING TO BE UP ALL NIGHT

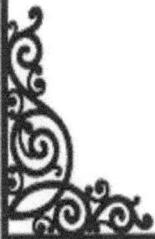

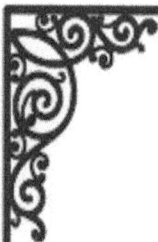

My yoga partner
is an egocentric
philanthropist.

After 10 years of
intensive yoga training,
he willed his
body to science...

But science is contesting
the will.

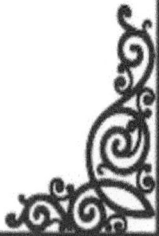

YOGA TEACHER TO LATE ARRIVING STUDENT:

TEACHER: "THIS IS THE FIFTH TIME YOU'VE BEEN LATE FOR CLASS THIS WEEK. DO YOU KNOW WHAT THAT MEANS?"

YOGA STUDENT: "THAT IT'S FRIDAY?"

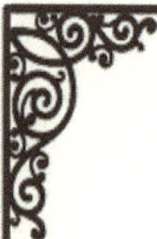

A YOGA INSTRUCTOR
CRITIQUES ONE OF HIS STUDENTS:

"SHE DOESN'T DO YOGA VERY
WELL...

I COMPARE HER TECHNIQUE
TO THAT OF AN ANGEL
WHO'S AFRAID OF HEIGHTS
AND CAN'T STAND
HARP MUSIC."

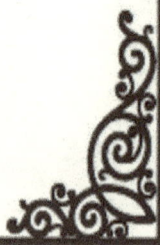

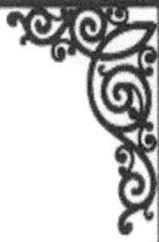

My yoga training goal
is not going well...

I took yoga to get back
to my original weight...

Eight pounds three ounces

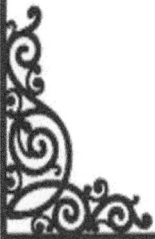

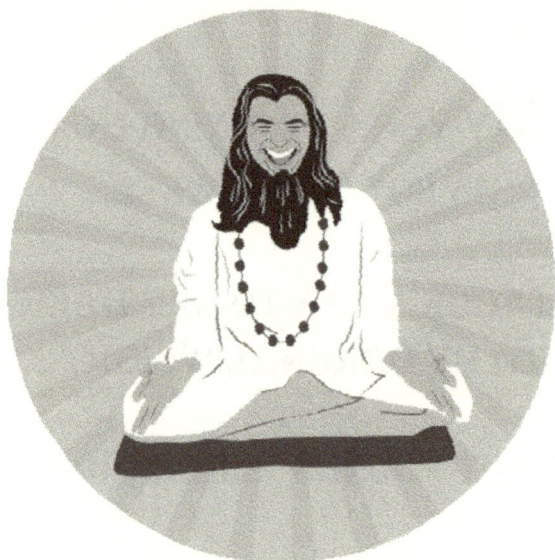

CHAPTER 12

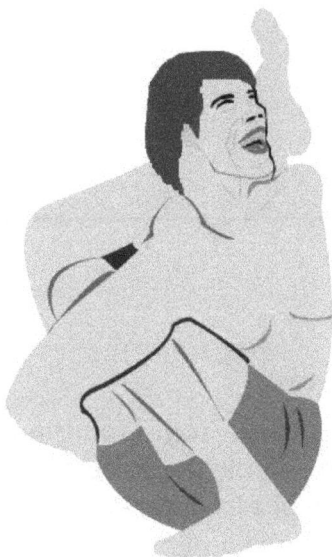

MARICHI ASANA
"Dedicated Twist Pose"

"The most important pieces of equipment you need for doing Yoga are your body and your mind."

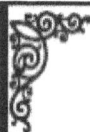

YOGA FACT:

The lotus pose in Yoga is a sitting pose meant to resemble the perfect symmetry and beauty of a lotus flower. Siddhartha Gautama, the founder of Buddhism, and Shiva, a major god in Hinduism, are typically shown in this pose.

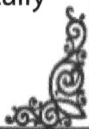

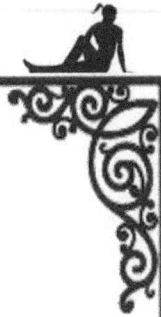

You know you really need
a yoga fitness class
when you can
pinch an inch...

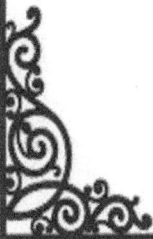

on your forehead.

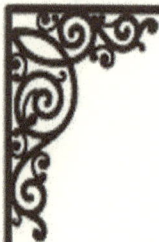

I'm on a strict yoga exercize program...

I started yesterday and I've only missed one day so far.

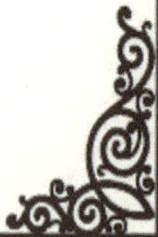

My teacher says i'm
a model yoga student...

but unfortunately,
not a working model.

My husband is overweight and doesn't do yoga.

He's attached to a machine that keeps him alive...

The refrigerator.

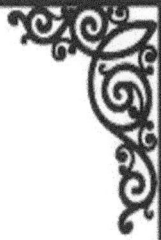

Yoga pupil asks the maharishi:

PUPIL: "WHAT WILL HAPPEN TO MEN IF GOD TURNS OUT TO BE A WOMAN?"

MAHARISHI: "NOT ONLY WILL WE ALL GO TO HELL, BUT WE'LL NEVER KNOW WHY."

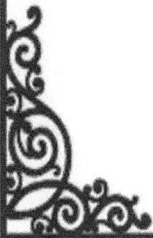

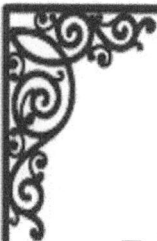

Yoga philosophy encourages us to be vegetarians.

I disagree with that thinking.

My ancestors didn't spend two million years to fight their way to the top of the food chain to be vegetarians.

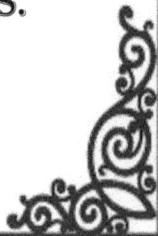

THE WISDOM OF THE MAHARISHI:

EVERYWHERE IS WITHIN WALKING DISTANCE...

IF YOU HAVE THE TIME.

Yoga philosophy teaches:

TO ATTAIN ENLIGHTENMENT...

YOU MUST REGULARLY
BREATHE IN,
AND BREATHE OUT.

FORGET THIS...

AND ATTAINING
ENLIGHTENMENT
WILL BE THE LEAST OF
YOUR PROBLEMS.

A VISITING YOGA STUDENT TO A POSH AND EXCLUSIVE BEVERLY HILLS ASHRAM ASKED ANOTHER STUDENT WHY EVERYBODY CURTSIED WHEN GREETING THE CELEBRITY YOGA TEACHER.

STUDENT: "CURTSY? HELL! IT'S A REQUIRED POSE FOR HIS CLASS...

WE'RE ONLY TRYING TO KISS HIS RING!"

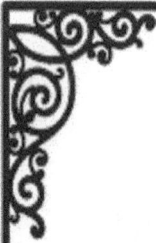

The Yoga pupil asks the guru:

Why have there been no romantic songs written about Yoga mats?

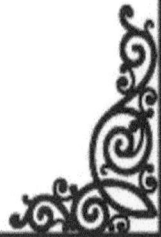

I PASSED UP A LOT OF
SINCERE AND
TALENTED YOGA TEACHERS
TO GET TO THE ONE
I FINALLY ENDED UP WITH.

A MAN BUYS A HOT DOG
FROM THE YOGI VENDOR
IN CENTRAL PARK:

THE PRICE ON THE CART SAYS
$5.00. HE TAKES THE HOT DOG
AND HANDS THE VENDOR A
$20 BILL. THE VENDOR
THANKS HIM AND CONTINUES
ROLLING HIS CART.

THE MAN SAYS...
"HEY, WHERE'S MY CHANGE?"

THE YOGI TURNS
AROUND AND SAYS...

"CHANGE MUST COME
FROM WITHIN."

A MAN GOES UP TO THE SAME $5 YOGI HOT DOG VENDOR IN CENTRAL PARK. THE MAN HANDS THE VENDOR A $20.00 BILL AND RECEIVES HIS HOT DOG. THE VENDOR POCKETS THE MONEY AND CONTINUES TO ROLL HIS CART DOWN THE STREET.

THE MAN, PUZZLED AND CONFUSED, HOLLERS OUT TO THE VENDOR, "HEY, WHAT ABOUT MY CHANGE?"

THE VENDOR TURNS AROUND AND SAYS, "IF YOU WANT CHANGE, SIGN UP FOR MY YOGA CLASS... YOU'LL GET CHANGE!"

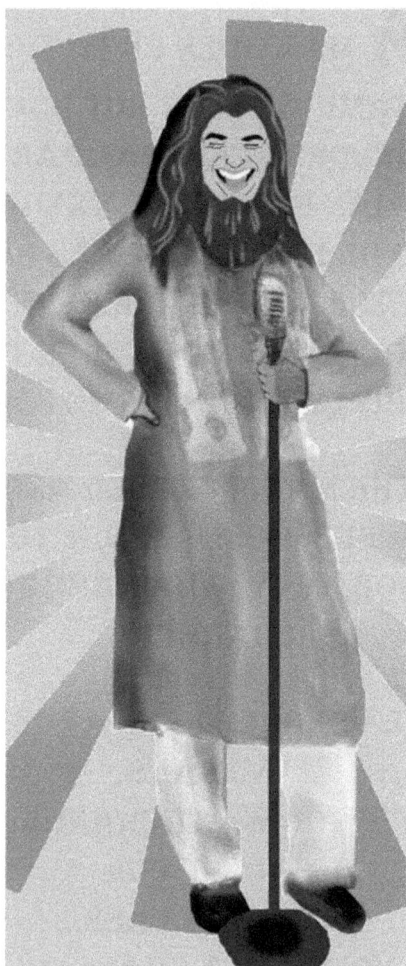

CHAPTER 13

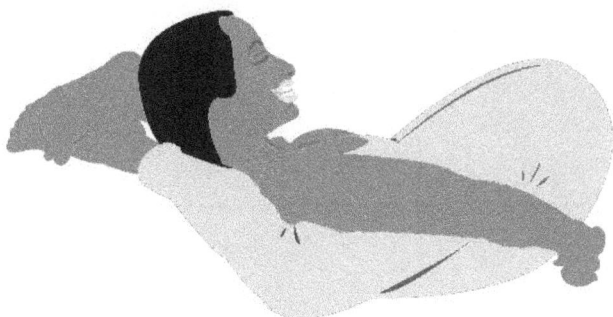

YOGANI ASANA
"Yogic Sleep Pose"

"Yoga will transform what has been a hindrance in your life into a teacher of the heart."

PHILLIP MOFFITT

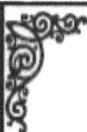

YOGA FACT:

Patanjali (150 B.C.), an Indian teacher, is considered to be the founder of Scientific Yoga and today's modern Yoga studies.

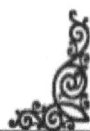

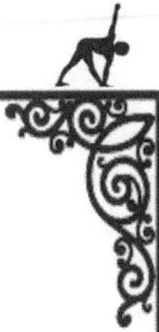

Yoga t-shirt:

Life is something that happens to you when you're not in yoga class.

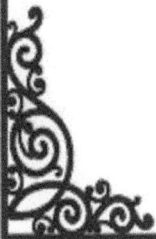

THE ONLY EXERCISE
I GET IN YOGA CLASS IS
BENDING TO MY
INSTRUCTOR'S WILL.

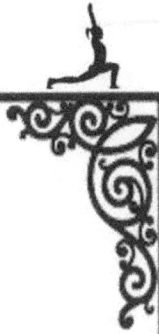

I WAS A PRETTY BAD YOGA
STUDENT...

I STOPPED GOING TO MY YOGA
CLASS FOR A WEEK AND GOT
A THANK YOU NOTE
FROM THE CLASS.

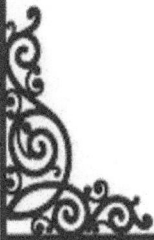

A BEVERLY HILLS YOGINI PROCLAIMS:

"I AM A YOGA PRINCESS...

FROM MY SEQUIN HEADBAND RIGHT DOWN TO MY GLASS SNEAKERS & MY ENCHANTED LEOTARDS."

It must be great to be
the maharishi.

You call up "Dial a Prayer"
and ask,

"Do I have any messages?"

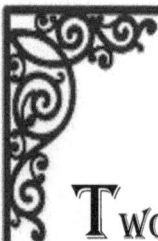

Two cats are carefully watching their owners doing their daily yoga workouts.

One cat, confused, shakes his head and says to the other,

"These guys are not very flexible. They've been doing their yoga training for over 10 years now, and they still can't lick their own behinds."

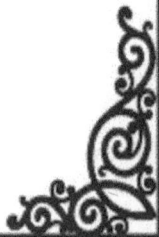

AT AN MORNING
ASHRAM CLASS LECTURE,
THE GURU ASKS HIS
AUDIENCE:

GURU: "HOW MANY OF YOU WOULD
LIKE TO GO TO NIRVANA?"

EVERYONE RAISED THEIR HANDS
EXCEPT FOR A YOUNG BLONDE
WOMAN SITTING IN THE FRONT
ROW.

GURU: "DON'T YOU WANT TO GO
TO NIRVANA?"

WOMAN: "YES, I'D LIKE TO GO,
BUT I'VE GOT MY
YOGA CLASS AT 3:00.

Sign on sleeping yogi monk in tibetan mountains:

"OUT OF BODY...
WILL BE BACK IN 15
MINUTES."

HAVE YOU EVER NOTICED THAT THE YOGA INSTRUCTOR SMILES MORE THAN THE STUDENTS?

An ex Yoga student speaks:

"I quit Yoga because of
illness & fatigue...

My teacher was
sick & tired of me."

Q. **H**OW MANY YOGIS DOES
IT TAKE TO
CHANGE A LIGHTBULB?

A. JUST ONE ...
BUT THEY REALLY
MUST WANT TO CHANGE.

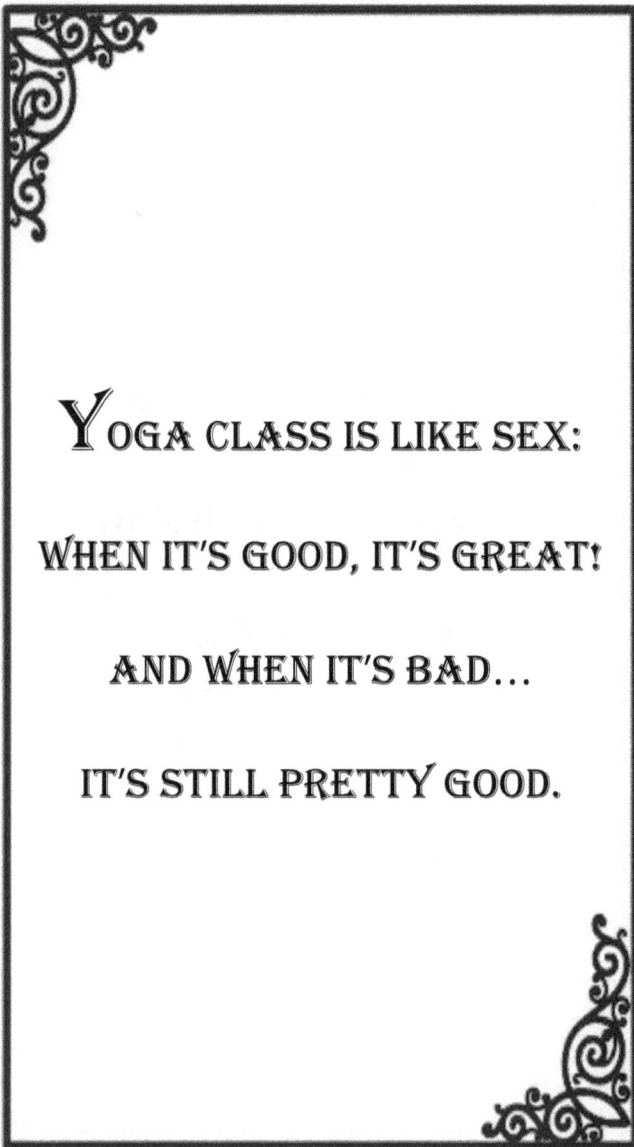

Yoga class is like sex:

when it's good, it's great!

and when it's bad…

it's still pretty good.

SIGN ON ASHRAM
BUILDING WINDOW:

PSYCHICS WANTED.
(YOU KNOW WHERE TO APPLY)

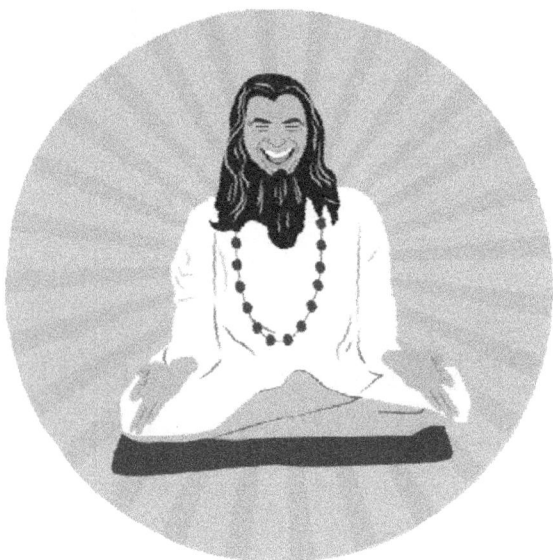

CHAPTER 14

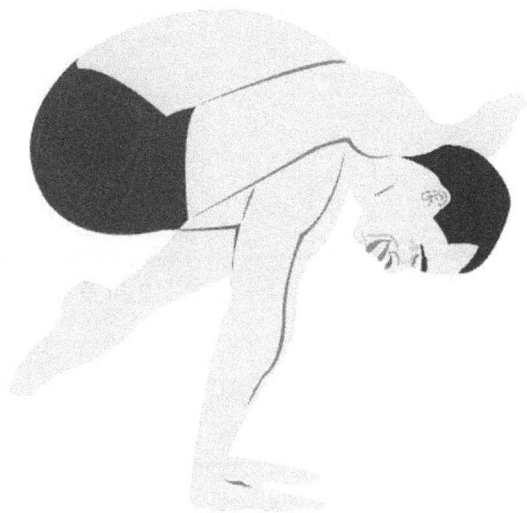

EKA PADA SIRSA BAK ASANA
"Behind The Head Crane Pose"

"Yoga is 99% practice and 1% theory."
SRI KRISHNA PATTABHI JOIS

YOGA FACT:

Swiss psychiatrist Carl Jung was one of the first Westerners to study Yoga in depth. His comments on developing higher consciousness in the East helped introduce the West to Yoga concepts and practices.

The yoga police say:

Bad Yoga technique
is not a crime...

So, you're free to go.

A MISSISSIPPI FARMER SPEAKS:

"AS FAR AS I'M CONCERNED,
YOGA IS FOR PEOPLE

WHO DON'T KNOW
HOW TO BOWL."

SENSITIVE MALE
YOGA TEACHERS
ARE LIKE UFOs...

YOU OFTEN HEAR
ABOUT THEM...

BUT NO ONE HAS
EVER SEEN ONE.

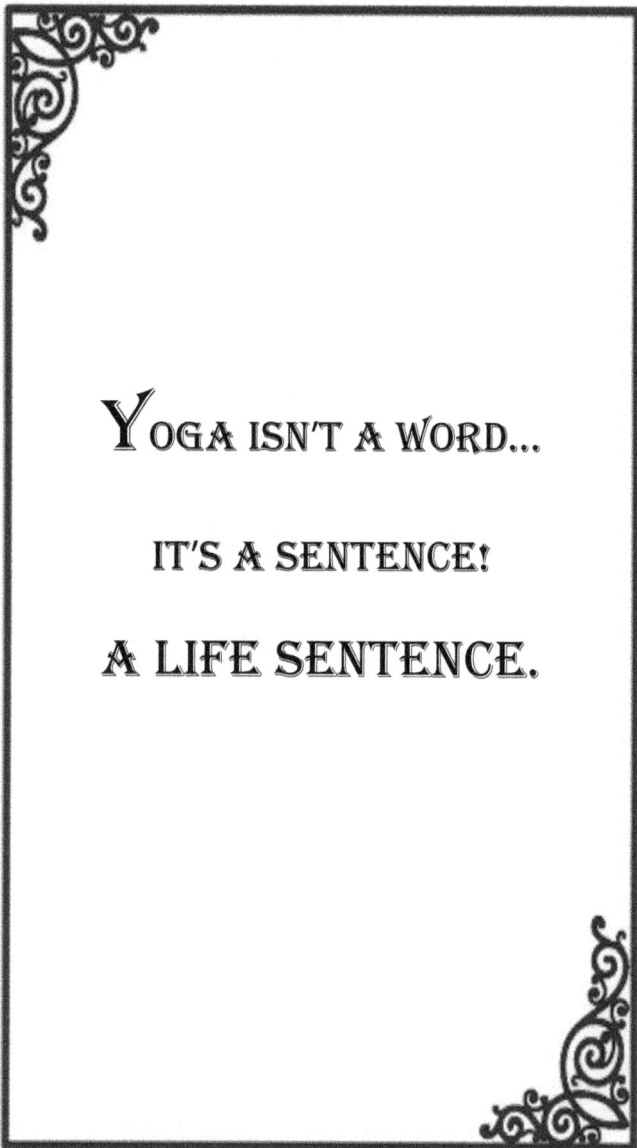

Yoga isn't a word...

It's a sentence!

A life sentence.

Two meditating yogis
meet on a pathway in
the himalayayas...

The first one says
to the other:

"You are fine. How am i?"

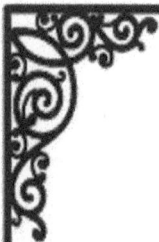

YOGA!
SEX!
FOOD!

WHAT ELSE IS THERE?

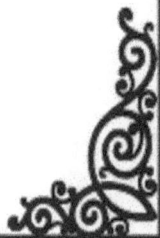

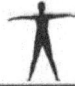

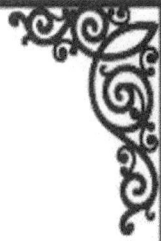

Before yoga,
My personal exercise routine was:

STRETCHING THE TRUTH
JOGGING MY MEMORY
PUSHING MY LUCK
JUMPING TO CONCLUSIONS

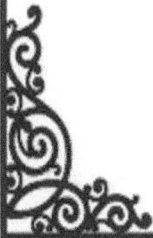

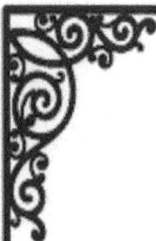

Yogini prayer:

Dear Lord:
If you can't make me skinny...

Please make my friends fat.

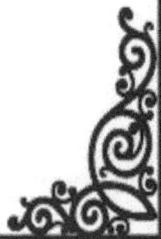

Two yoginis are talking at the ashram...

1ST YOGINI: "HOW'S YOUR HUSBAND GETTING ALONG WITH HIS YOGA TRAINING? IS HE IMPROVING HIS TECHNIQUE?"

2ND YOGINI: MUCH BETTER. IN FACT, HE'S IMPROVED TO THE POINT WHERE THE CHILDREN ARE NOW ALLOWED TO WATCH HIM DO HIS ASANAS."

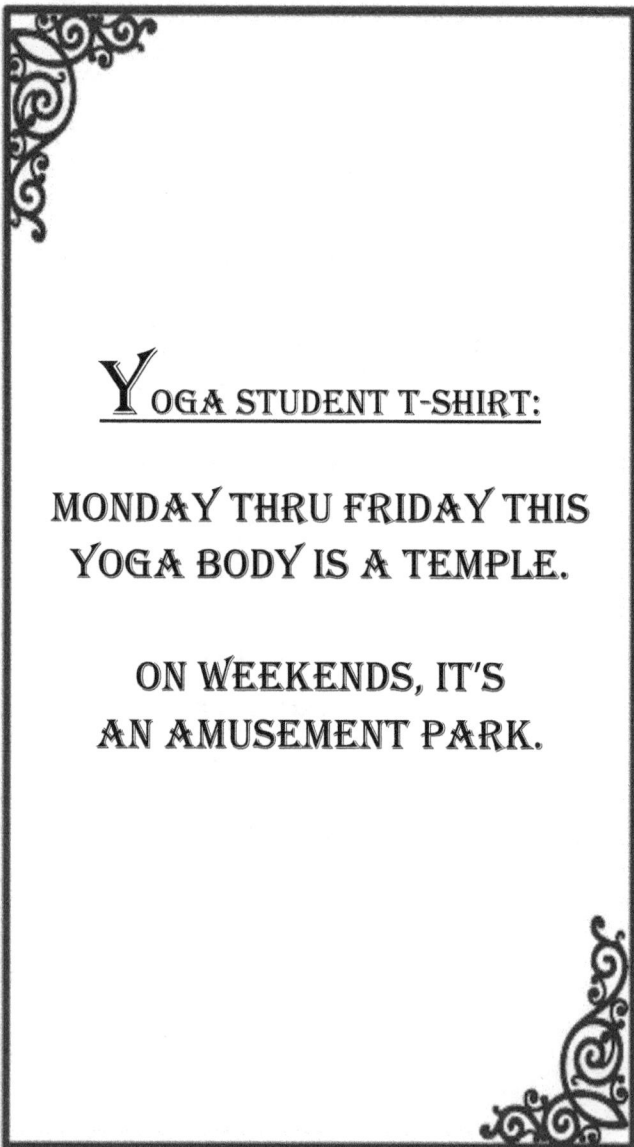

Yoga student t-shirt:

Monday thru Friday this Yoga body is a temple.

On weekends, it's an amusement park.

Man cannot live by yoga alone!

that's why god created chocolate.

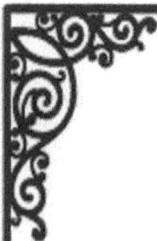

SOME YOGA PEOPLE LIKE
DOING THE 'DOWNWARD DOG'
AND THE 'COBRA' POSES...

BUT I HAVE MY OWN FAVORITE
NON-YOGA POSES:

"THE REFRIGERATOR LUNGE"
FOLLOWED BY
"THE MICROWAVE PUSH."

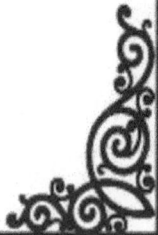

At a funeral where the casket was open, a woman walked by and gazed inside at the body of a 25-year old yoga student. She said to one of the mourners:

FIRST WOMAN: "HE LOOKS TERRIFIC."

SECOND WOMAN: "WHY SHOULDN'T HE? FOR THE LAST MONTH, HE DID HOT YOGA THREE TIMES A DAY."

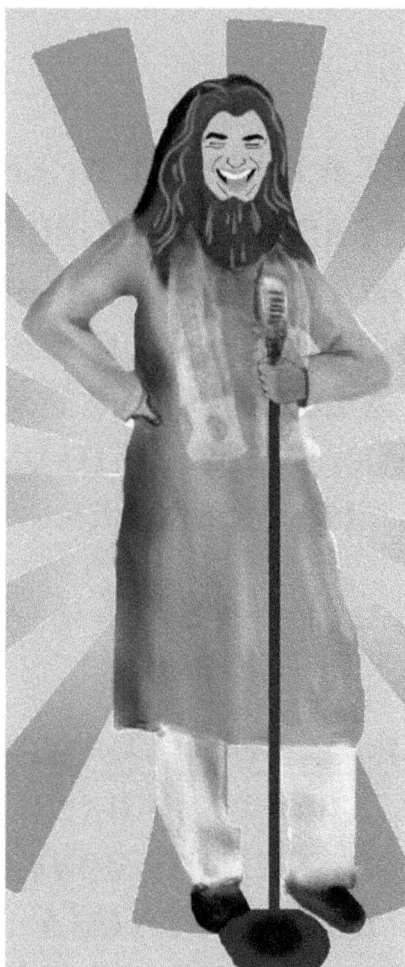

CHAPTER 15

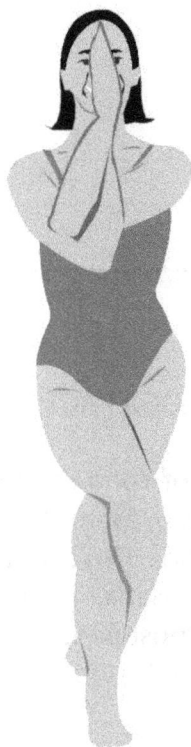

GARUD ASANA
"Eagle Pose"

"For me, Yoga is not just a workout; it's about working on yourself."

MARY GLOVER

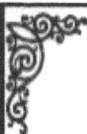

YOGA FACT:

Patanjali's 8 steps of Yoga is defined as follows:
Yama, Niyama, Asana, Pranayama,
Pratyhara, Dharana, Dhyana, and Samadhi.
The third step, "Asana," refers to postures
and poses that most people think of when
they hear the word "Yoga."

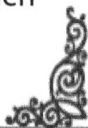

WISDOM OF THE MAHARISHI:

"WHEN AN 84-YEAR-OLD YOGI MARRIES AN 80-YEAR-OLD YOGINI, DON'T THROW RICE AT THE WEDDING...

THROW VIAGRA."

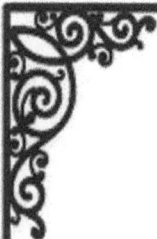

An elderly yoga student says:

"Despite what my yoga teachings tell me, I still won't eat organic foods...

At my age, I need all the preservatives I can get.

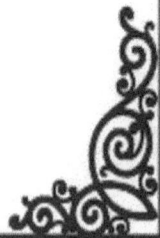

MEN LIKE TO DATE THIN
YOGINIS BECAUSE THEY'RE
TOO WEAK TO ARGUE...

AND SALADS ARE CHEAP.

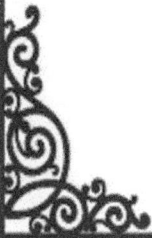

My wife finally got
me motivated
to do Yoga sit ups...

She put the remote
control between
my toes.

Q. **W**HAT DOES YOGA
MEDITATION AND AN
APPLE PEELER HAVE
IN COMMON?

A. THEY BOTH TAKE YOU
TO THE CORE.

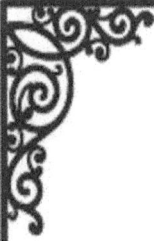

GRAFITTI ON THE ASHRAM WALL:

IS DOGMA
THE MOTHER
OF ALL DOGS?

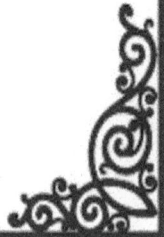

Swami's advice
for new yoga students:

IF YOU THINK IT'S HARD TO
MEET NEW PEOPLE AT YOUR
ASHRAM CLASS...

JUST TRY PICKING UP
SOMEONE ELSE'S YOGA MAT.

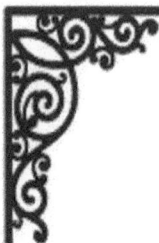

Yoga reincarnation philosophy says:

My body will come back to life after I die...

So, why am I exercising to keep this one in shape?

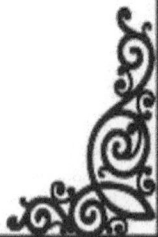

Yoga confuses me...

I don't know what
I need more:

To pull myself together
or to let myself go?

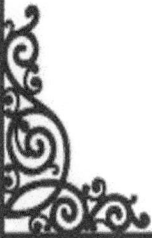

Q. How many new hatha yoga students does it take to change a light bulb?

A. Only one...

But they'll need four blankets, a chair, six blocks, and two straps to do it.

THERE ARE FOUR THINGS
I WANT IN LIFE...

1. HOT YOGA WORKOUTS.
2. HAPPINESS.
3. SEX.
4. CHOCOLATE.

BUT NOT NECESSARILY IN
THAT ORDER.

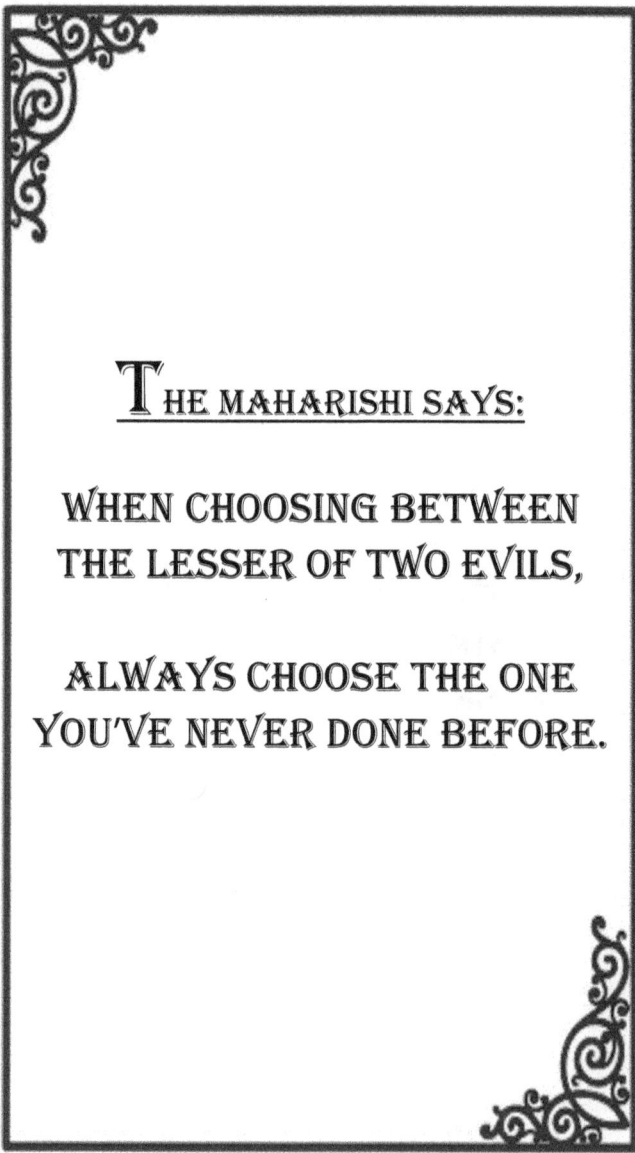

The maharishi says:

When choosing between the lesser of two evils,

always choose the one you've never done before.

DOING YOGA
DOESN'T MEAN
YOU'LL LIVE LONGER...

IT WILL JUST SEEM LONGER.

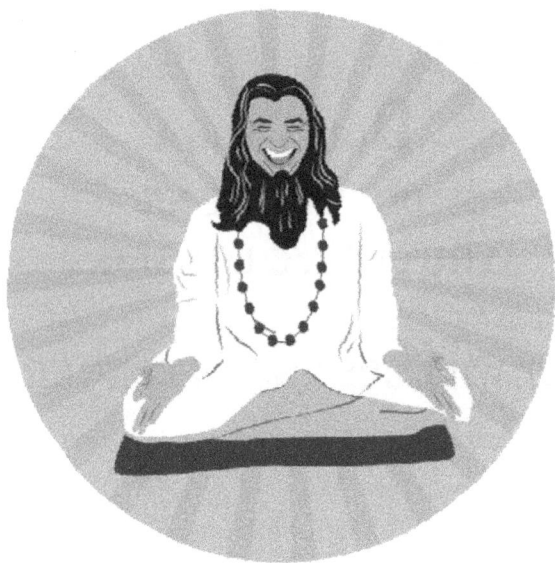

CHAPTER 16

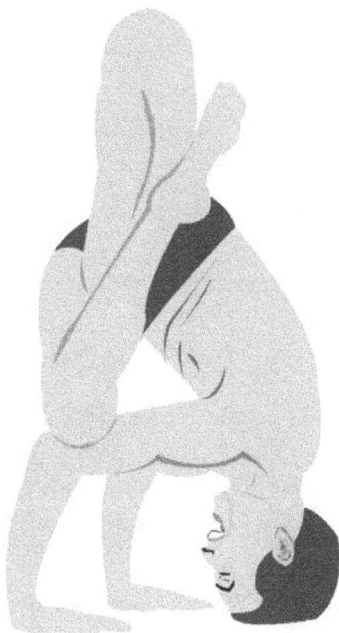

PARSVA KUKKIT ASANA
"The Side Roost Pose"

"Yoga is the practice of quieting the mind."
<u>PATANJALI</u>

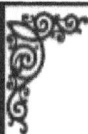

YOGA FACT:

"Doga" is a type of Yoga in which people use Yoga to achieve harmony with their pets. Dogs can either be used as props for their owners or they can do the stretches themselves. It reportedly started in New York in 2002 when Suzi Teitelman started "Yoga for Dogs."

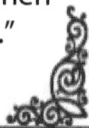

AN EX-YOGA STUDENT SAYS:

THERE'S A FINE LINE BETWEEN DOING ASANAS...

AND JUST SITTING IN A YOGA CLASS LOOKING LIKE AN IDIOT

Two little girls were looking at the scale in their Yogini mother's bathroom.

One little girl warns her friend:

"Don't step on that thing, it makes you cry."

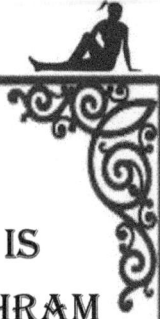

An instructor is talking to the ashram owner about their wealthy 86 year old student:

INSTRUCTOR: "I think she is getting too old for yoga training."

OWNER: "Why do you say that?"

INSTRUCTOR: Because she has to have two boy scouts help her complete each asana."

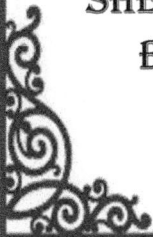

Setting the record straight:

Yogi bear is not an instructor at the jellystone park ashram.

A NEW YOGA STUDENT SPEAKS:

"I HAD TO GIVE UP ATHEISM WHEN I BEGAN MY YOGA TRAINING.

I HAD NO CHOICE...

WHEN YOU DO YOGA AS BAD AS I DO, YOU'VE GOT TO HAVE SOMEONE TO PRAY TO."

Yoga philosophy:

Inside every overweight
yoga student,
there's a thin person
screaming to get out...

But usually you can quiet
them down with four or
five Snicker's bars.

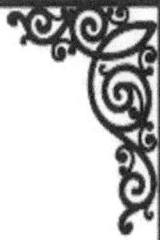

THE GURU SAYS:

OUR UNIVERSE IS MADE
UP OF PROTONS,
NEUTRONS
AND
ELECTRONS.

HE FORGOT TO MENTION
MORONS.

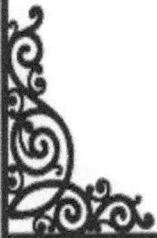

A YOGINI SPEAKS:

DESPITE MY YOGA TEACHINGS, I DO NOT BELIEVE IN AN AFTER LIFE.

BUT I'M NOT TAKING ANY CHANCES EITHER...

BECAUSE WHEREVER I GO, I ALWAYS TAKE AN EXTRA YOGA MAT AND PAIR OF LEOTARDS WITH ME

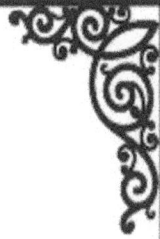

Maharishi wisdom:

NEVER ARGUE WITH
A YOGINI WHEN
SHE'S TIRED....

OR WHEN SHE'S RESTED.

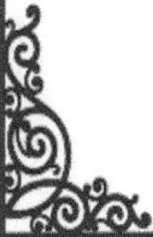

The majority of U.S. Yoga instructors agree that there are 3 rules for perfecting your Yoga training...

Unfortunately, they won't tell anyone what they are.

YOGA CONFUSES ME.

BECAUSE...

IF PRACTICE MAKES PERFECT,
AND NO ONE IS PERFECT,

THEN WHY PRACTICE?

When I was a boy my yogini mother wore a mystic color mood ring...

When she was in a good mood, it turned blue.

And when she was in a bad mood...

It left a big, red mark on my forehead.

THE PUPIL ASKS THE GURU:

IF YOU HAVE AN AFFAIR WITH
YOUR YOGA TEACHER,
WOULD THAT PUT YOU IN
A DIFFICULT POSITION?

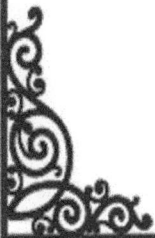

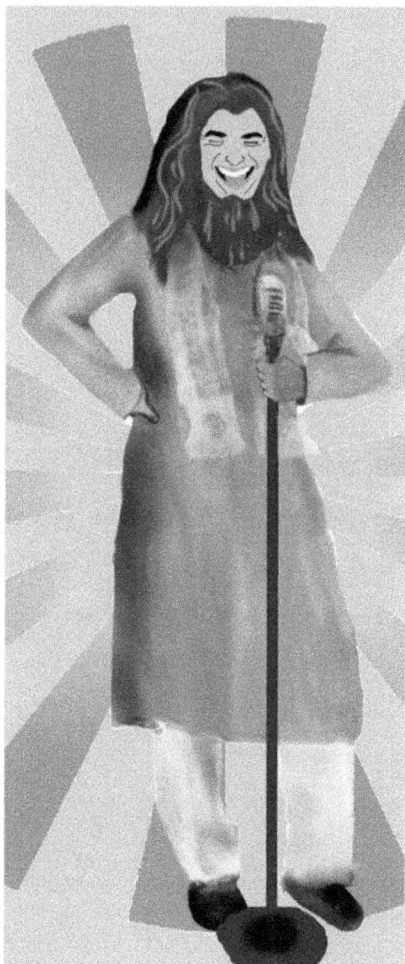

CHAPTER 17

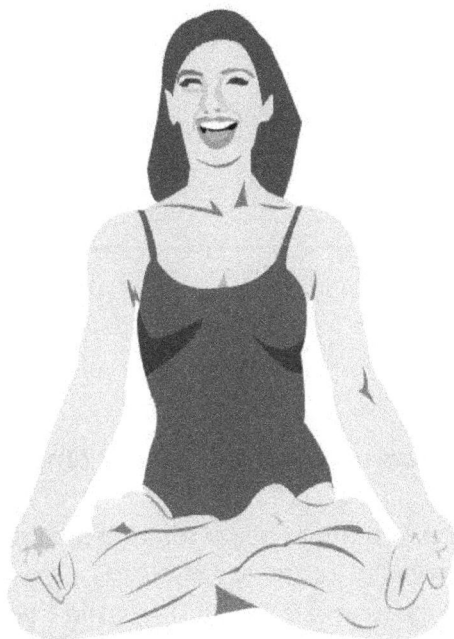

TRIKAKONA ASANA
"3 Point Stance" (Meditation Pose)

"Yoga accepts. Yoga gives."

APRIL VALLEI

YOGA FACT:

Scholars note that just as the computer scientists who built ARPANET (the early Internet) created the conditions for Google, so American transcendentalist Ralph Waldo Emerson (1803-1882) created the conditions for American Yoga.

THE NEW L.A. STUDENT'S
YOGA OUTFITS ARE FASHION
CREATIONS THAT WILL NEVER
GO OUT OF STYLE...

THEY WILL LOOK JUST AS
RIDICULOUS
YEAR AFTER YEAR.

Some undertakers endorse the Yoga belief in reincarnation...

Why not?

It's a chance for repeat business.

The one good thing yoga teaches us about reincarnation...

Is that you don't have to bring much luggage.

Our tuesday night Yoga instructor, Mr. Berkley, talks so much and holds our poses so long that we finally had to have a serious discussion with him...

We said; "Mr. Berkley, the reason we call it 'Tuesday night class' is because it's supposed to begin and end on the same day."

During a pre-class warm-up, a muscular yoga student couldn't keep his eyes off the good-looking, sexy yogini doing her asanas on the floor.

He turns to the instructor and asks:

STUDENT: "What pose can I do to impress her?"

INSTRUCTOR: "There's only one... 'The Credit Card Swipe at Tiffany's Pose.'

I DO 10 YOGA SIT-UPS
EVERY MORNING...

IT MIGHT NOT SOUND LIKE
A LOT, BUT THERE ARE ONLY
SO MANY TIMES YOU CAN HIT
THE SNOOZE BUTTON.

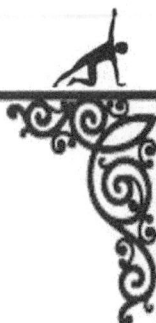

I DO MY YOGA EXERCISES
RELIGIOUSLY...

I PERFORM ONE
YOGA HEADSTAND
AND I SAY,
"AMEN!"

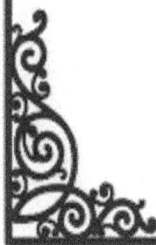

THE RELIGIOUS HUSBAND
OF A VERY ACTIVE
YOGA STUDENT, MEETS HER
INSTRUCTOR ON THE STREET.
HE ASKS HIM:

HUSBAND: "IS IT WRONG FOR
MY WIFE TO PRACTICE HER
YOGA ON SUNDAYS?"

INSTRUCTOR: "I'VE SEEN YOUR
WIFE PRACTICE, AND, BELIEVE
ME, THE WAY SHE DOES YOGA,
IT'S WRONG ANY
DAY OF THE WEEK!

Two women are talking in the ashram;

FIRST WOMAN: "SURELY, YOU CAN'T BELIEVE YOUR HUSBAND'S STORY THAT HE WENT OUT OF TOWN TO ENTER A YOGA TOURNAMENT IN LAS VEGAS? ... AND IF YOU NOTICED, HE DIDN'T BRING BACK ANY TROPHIES OR RIBBONS.

SECOND WOMAN: THAT'S WHAT MADE ME BELIEVE HE WAS REALLY COMPETING IN A YOGA TOURNAMENT.

Q. Do female students
sleep with their yoga
teachers?

A. No, they make love to
them.

They sleep with their
husbands.

Q. **W**HERE DOES A
400 POUND YOGA STUDENT
TRAIN IN THE ASHRAM?

A. ANYWHERE HE
DAMN WELL WANTS TO!

Ex yoga student speaks:

"For me the second day of yoga class was easier than the first...

Because on the second day, I quit!"

I HAVE TO DO MY YOGA
EXERCISES EARLY
IN THE MORNING...

BEFORE MY BRAIN FIGURES
OUT WHAT I'M DOING.

Yoga:

A NEW STUDENT'S DEFINITION:

"A SERIES OF
STRENUOUS EXERCISES
WHICH HELP CONVERT
FATS, SUGARS
AND STARCHES
INTO
ACHES, PAINS
AND CRAMPS."

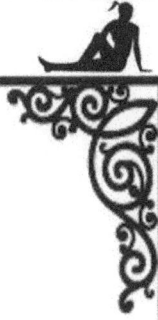

YOU KNOW YOU NEED A YOGA WEIGHT LOSS PROGRAM...

WHEN YOUR STOMACH IS PUSHING YOUR SOCKS DOWN.

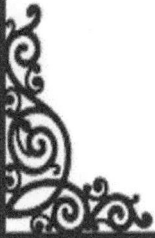

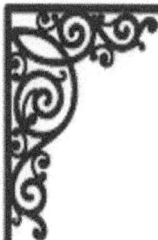

Yoga teacher t-shirt:

I don't suffer from Yoga stress.

I am a carrier.

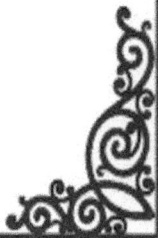

A NEW STUDENT SPEAKS:

I WAS A LITTLE CONFUSED
WHEN I FIRST STARTED
YOGA TRAINING.

MY TEACHER TOLD ME THAT
I COULD HAVE THE BODY OF
AN 18-YEAR-OLD...

BUT WHERE WOULD I KEEP IT?

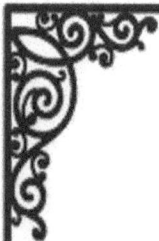

I WENT TO ONE OF THOSE
YOGA HEALTH-FOOD
RESTAURANTS
AND WAS AMAZED...

EVEN THE FLIES WERE DOING
THE WARRIOR POSE.

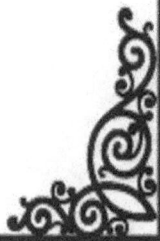

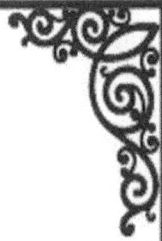

My grandmother is very much into yoga and fitness.

She started walking 5 miles a day when she was 50. She's 78 now...

And we don't know where the hell she is.

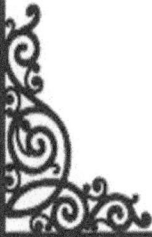

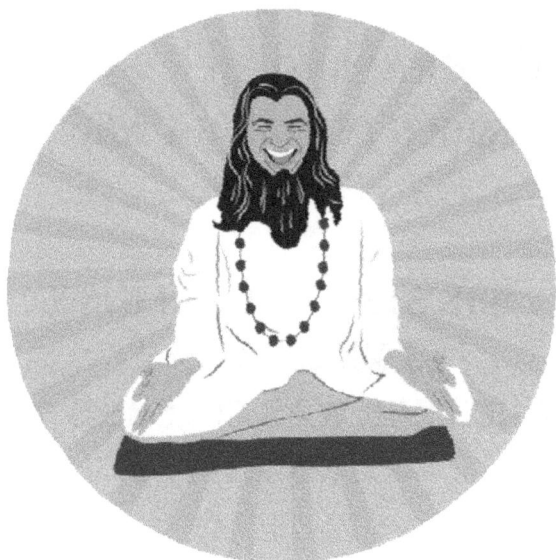

YOGA LAFFS GLOSSARY

ACUPUNCTURE: An Ancient Far Eastern Healing Technique Where Needle Pressure is Applied to a Particular Nerve, Stimulating Healing to a Certain Area of the Body.

ASANA: A Yoga Pose or Posture Utilized in Hatha Yoga.

ASHRAM: A Place of Study. Unique to Yoga and the Various Approaches to Mind, Body and Breath Disciplines.

ASHTANGA YOGA: 8 Limbed Scientific Yoga Training Study.

ATTACHMENTS: Identifying With Anything That Limits You, in Particular; Those Things of Pain and Pleasure.

BIHAR YOGA: Also Known As "Yoga Therapy"— A Study That Emphasizes Breathing, Chanting and Asanas.

BIKRAM YOGA: See "Hot Yoga."

"COBRA ASANA": A Yoga Pose Focusing on the Spine.

CORE: The Bodily Center of an Asana Movement.

DHYANA YOGA: Meditation Yoga Developed in Ancient India.

DOGMA: An Authoritative Doctrine, Philosophy or Belief Proclaimed as Unquestionably True By a Particular Group or Individuals.

"DOWNWARD DOG ASANA: A Yoga Posture, Lengthening the Back and the Legs.

DWI PADASIRS ASANA: "Behind The Head Pose" (See Page 49); To Develop Continuing Balance and Hip Flexibility.

EKA PADA SIRSA BAK ASANA: "One Foot Behind the Head Crane Pose" (See Page 209); To Develop Balance and Strength.

EMPOWERMENT: To Give Yourself or Others the Power, Authority or Permission to Complete a Certain Task or Mission.

ENLIGHTENMENT: Liberation or Self-Realization; "Seeing All Things Clearly."

GARUD ASANA: "Eagle Pose" (See Page 225); To Develop Balance and Alignment.

GARUD ASANA IN SIRS ASANA: "Headstand With Eagle Legs" (See Page 81); To Develop Balance and Encourage Reverse Circulation.

GURU: A Yoga Teacher.

HATHA YOGA (HA/SUN) (THA/MOON): One of the Eight Limbs of Yoga Study Through Asanas.

"HOT YOGA" (BIKRAM YOGA): Modern Yoga Technique Created/Developed by the Guru Bikram of Beverly Hills, California. A Technique Created To Be Practiced in Heat, Combined With Breathing and Profuse Sweating.

IYENGAR YOGA: A Popular School of Yoga that Emphasizes Precise Alignment of Each Yoga Asana, Created by the Modern Indian Guru, Iyengar.

JIVA MUKTI YOGA: A Chanting Yoga of Flowing non-stop Asanas.

KARMA: The Force Generated by a Person's Actions Which Determines Ones Destiny, Good or Bad, Either in This Life or in Reincarnation.

KUNDALINI YOGA: The Study of Yoga Empathizing the Body's Energy Through the Spine.

MAHARISHI: A Great Spiritual Leader with Followers.

MANTRA: Vocal Sounds of Empowerment. Can be a Single Sound or Many Sounds.

MARICHY ASANA: "Dedicated Twist Pose" (See Page 177); To Develop the Skill of the Opposite Limbs Through the Core.

MEDITATION: Inward Study and Observation of One's Self Through the Study of Yoga.

METAPHYSICS: An Ancient Approach to Understanding and Solving of Something Cosmic or Every Day Living.

MONK: A Student of a Particular Religious Study

NATARA JASANA: "Dance Pose" (See Page 161); To Develop Balance and Spinal Flexibility.

NIRALAMBA SIRSASANA: "Unsupported Headstand" (See Page 65); To Develop Reverse Circulation and Upward Development of the Core.

NIRVANA: An Sanskrit term used to describe the freeing of one from all that enslaves it. The happiness that comes when all passion, hatred and delusion die out. It is the peace of mind and freedom that is *moshka* (liberation) and union with the Supreme Being.

PADMA VIPARITASALABHASANA: "Locust Pose" (See Page 17); To Develop Shoulder Strength Through the Core.)

PARSVA KUKIKT ASANA: "The Side Roost Pose" (See Page 241); To Develop Reverse Circulation, Core Alignment and Shoulder Strength.

PRANAYAMA YOGA: Breathing and Energy Studies and Exercises.

PRESENCE: In Yoga, a Training Tradition of "Being There" in what is Taking Place at a Given Moment

REINCARNATION: An ancient Indian Belief That You Will Return to Life in One Form or Another Based on Your Karma.

SANSKRIT: The Classical Language of Ancient India.

SIDDH ASANA: "Lotus Adapt Pose" (See Page 1); To Develop Reflection, Calmness and Perfect Symmetry.

SIVANDA YOGA: Yoga Study Based on Chanting and Breathing Techniques.

SUN As/SUN Bs: A Choreographed Set of Yoga Asanas.

SWAMI: Spiritual Teacher and Leader.

TRANSCIDENTAL MEDITATION: A Modern Approach to Meditation Made Popular by Various Celebrities in 1960's.

TRIKAKONA ASANA: "3-Point Stance" Meditation Pose (see page 257); To Develop Reflection, Calmness and Perfect Symmetry.

URDHVA PRASARITA EKS PAD ASANA: "One Legged Forward Bend Pose" (See Page 129); Develops the Lengthening of the Body from Head to Toe.

UTTHITATRIKON ASANA: "Extended Triangle Pose" (See Page 97); Develops Strength, Agility and Focus

VALGUL ASANA: "The Bat Pose" (See Page 145)

VEGETARIAN: Person(s) Who Only Eat Fruits, Vegetables, and Grains - No Meat.

VIRANCHY ASANA: "Dedicated Pose" (See Page 33)

VIRAVHADR ASANA: "The Warrior" (See Page 113)

VINI YOGA: A Gentle Yoga Study using Pranayama Breathing Techniques.

YOGA: Ancient Sanskrit Word Meaning "The Union." A Study of Mind, Body and Spirit Using a Series of Postures and Breathing Exercises Practiced to Achieve Control of the Body and Mind towards Tranquility.

YOGA MASTER: A Respected, Knowledgeable and Experienced Student and Teacher of the Study of Yoga.

YOGA MAT: A Cloth or Piece of Material That You Lay or Stand On During Yoga Training.

YOGANI DRASANA: "Yogic Sleep Pose." (See Page 193)

YOGI: A Male Yoga Student

YOGINI: A Female Yoga Student

"YOGA IS NOT A MATTER OF LIFE OR DEATH...

IT'S MORE IMPORTANT THAN THAT."

Laurence Berkley – Hatha Yoga Instructor

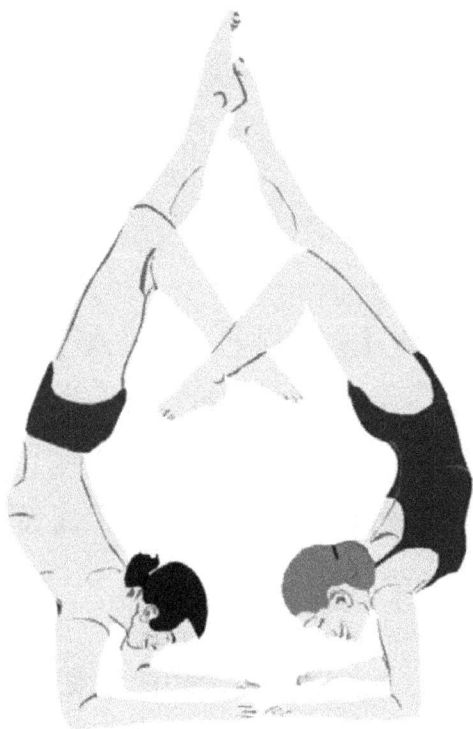

THE JOY OF YOGA

YOGA LAFFS

Original, Collectible Comedy Prints

All Signed, Numbered, & Ready To Frame

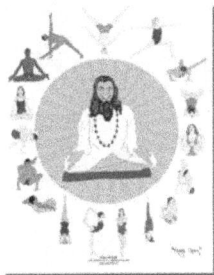

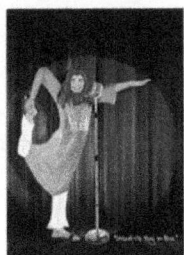

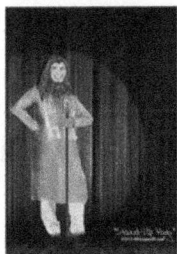

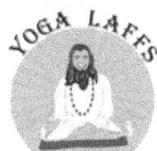

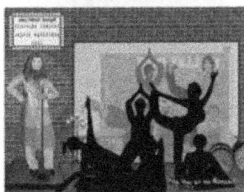

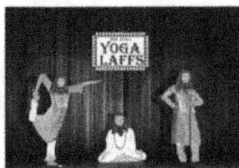

Full Color - 11"x14" Prints
Check Out All The Great Comedy Art At
www.YogaLaffs.com

CHECK OUT ALL THE LAUGHS AT
YOGALAFFS.COM

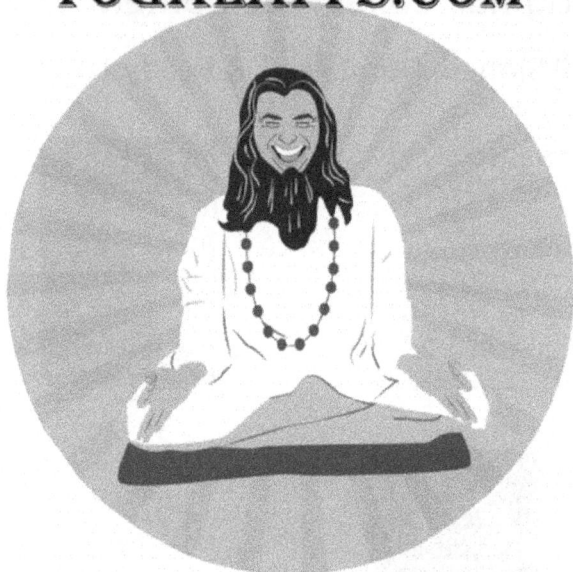

The Official Website for Yoga Laughter!

Share your funny Yoga jokes, stories, quotes, and comedic observations with Yoga Laffs. If we use them in our next book, we will send you a free copy of *Yoga Laffs 2*!

Enter your favorite Yoga Joke(s) at the Yoga Laffs website,

www.yogalaffs.com

Published by

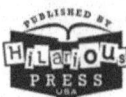